B. O. Hütter

Neuropsychological Sequelae of Subarachnoid Hemorrhage and its Treatment

With Forewords
by W. Seeger
and K. Poeck

SpringerWienNewYork

Priv.-Doz. Dipl.-Psych. Dr. phil. B.O. Hütter
Neurochirurgische Universitätsklinik,
RWTH Aachen, Germany

Printed in Austria

Typesetting: Scientific Publishing Services (P) Ltd., Madras
Printing and Binding: Manz Crossmedia, A-1051 Wien

Printed on acid-free and chlorine-free bleached paper

SPIN: 10711522

With 4 Figures

CIP data applied for

ISBN 3-211-83442-7 Springer-Verlag Wien New York

Foreword by Wolfgang Seeger

Neurosurgical outcome gradings usually divide the result of operative treatment into excellent, good, mild or severe deficits and lethal courses. Psychological changes were frequently overlooked or regarded only as a mild impairment. If one compares the frequency of preoperative psycho-organic syndromes as documented in the medical records with the results of sophisticated psychological testing procedures, it becomes evident that an unexpectedly large range of psychological disorders cannot be identified by means of a conventional clinical examination.

Therefore, among neurosurgeons in the last years there is a growing interest in the results of pre- and postoperative psychosomatic, psychopathological and neuropsychological investigations. This is additionally motivated by the need to differentiate illness-related from surgically induced defects as well as postoperative improvements. Physical damage such as the presence of a hemiparesis is clearly defined while non-psychologists are not so familiar with psychological changes. However, these invisible 'deficits' even if mild, are of substantial relevance for social adjustment when the patient is able to work. This becomes obvious if one resumes the social catamnesia of patients after cerebral damage marked by the rise of severe psychosocial maladjustment.

The author of this monograph has sought the scientific collaboration with neurosurgeons since he finished his academic training as a psychologist 10 years ago. From the beginning he has been particularly interested in the psychological sequelae of aneurysmal subarachnoid hemorrhage and its surgical treatment. As a first step of research, he tried to identify the sequelae of uni- and bilateral limbic damage related to the posterior parts of the gyrus rectus and the subcallosal area. It was logical to conduct the first studies on the neuropsychological consequences of the rupture and surgical repair of aneurysms of the anterior communicating artery, because this is the most frequent location of aneurysms, and the above-mentioned anatomical structures are closely related to it.

Surgical damage is frequently inevitable if the neurosurgeon prepares the neck of the aneurysm in order to clip it to prevent a new rupture. This element of surgical treatment has gained a new interest since the introduction of endovascular methods for eliminating intracranial aneurysms. The endovascular method may have the advantage not to damage the brain parenchyma if no inadvertent closure of perforating vessels close to the aneurysm occurs. Furthermore, the advent of MR tomography substantially improved the visualization of damage to the brain substance.

In earlier times the postoperative psychological changes were attributed to the local damage caused by aneurysm surgery. Meanwhile, in the age of modern microneurosurgery, this assumption cannot be upheld anymore.

The data about different aneurysm locations given in the present work clearly demonstrate that the quality and the severity of the neuropsychological impairments after subarachnoid hemorrhage are in particular dependent on the anatomical location and extent of the bleeding. In addition, the sometimes inevitable temporary clipping of perforating vessels seems to play a significant role with respect to later neuropsychological disturbances.

Since modern aneurysm surgery is performed in the acute phase shortly after the hemorrhage, the findings reported in the present work are, according to my opinion, of particular relevance. In the light of the present intensive discussion about the indication for microneurosurgical clipping or neuroradiological interventional coiling of intracranial aneurysms, the results given here in by B. O. Hütter can be regarded as an argument for the surgical intervention, in particular because the extravasated blood can only be cleared by surgery.

Therefore, this book may be an inspiration for the neurosurgical reader for a closer collaboration with psychologically trained scientists. This is important for all intracranial processes and not only for the topic of subarachnoid hemorrhage covered by this book.

Freiburg, November 1999 *Wolfgang Seeger*

Foreword by Klaus Poeck

For want of more refined instruments the outcome of neurosurgical patients is assessed mostly by means of the Glasgow Outcome Scale. This scale, however, does not reflect mild grades of cognitive impairment and, more important, psychosocial variables that have recently been termed health (or rather: sickness) related quality of life (QOL). Research into the QOL domain has been conducted mostly in an anecdotical way.

This monograph is a most valuable attempt to elucidate QOL in a well defined neurosurgical population, namely patients with subarachnoid hemorrhage (SAH) with and without surgery for aneurysms of various location and with clinical syndromes of different severity. With a view to operationalize a concept that is frequently considered as based on "soft" data, the author has developed an inventory that yields data in a controlled way, including self-report and relative-report on the patient's functioning and well-being. The stratification of patients permitted the separate assessment of the neurobehavioral consequences of bleeding and of bleeding plus surgery in relation to different aneurysm sites, mild and severe Hunt and Hess grades and, of course, the usual demographic variables.

The author has adduced a wealth of personal data, meticulously discussed against the background of the literature. The QOL findings will be of value for the neurosurgeon's decision making and serve as a rational basis for seeking the patient's informed consent. The broad scope of the monograph is highlighted by the final discussions on the extent to which patients experience SAH as a psychological trauma and on the possible impact of the reported findings on rehabilitation programs.

Aachen/Bonn, December 1999 *Klaus Poeck*

Acknowledgement

I acknowledge gratefully the assistance of Dr. I. Kreitschmann-Andermahr, Department of Neurosurgery, Medical Faculty of the RWTH Aachen, who translated the manuscript into English.

B. O. Hütter

Contents

List of abbreviations

A.	Arteria
AANS	American Association of Neurosurgeons
ACA	anterior cerebral artery
ACoA	anterior communicating artery
AICA	inferior anterior cerebellar artery
ALQI	Aachen Life Quality Inventory
AV-malformation	arterio-venous malformation
Babif	Basilar bifurcation
BDI	Beck Depression Inventory
BI	Barthel Index
CBF	cerebral blood flow
CCT	cranial computed tomography
C.	Cisterna
CNS	central nervous system
COPD	chronic obstructive pulmonary disease
CSF	cerebrospinal fluid
DSM-IV	Diagnostic and Statistical Manual for Classification of Mental Disorders, fourth edition
ECG	electrocardiogram
FPI-R	Freiburg Personality Inventory-Revised
FWIT	Color-Word-Interference task (Stroop test)
GCS	Glasgow Coma Scale
GOS	Glasgow Outcome Scale
HMPAO SPECT	Hydrogen-Phosphoroxyd-Single-Photon-Emission-Computed-Tomography
ICA	internal carotid artery
ICH	intracerebral hemorrhage
IES	Impact of Event Scale
IQ	intelligence quotient
IST	Intelligenz-Struktur-Test
IVH	intraventricular hemorrhage
LPS	Leistungsprüfsystem
MCA	medial cerebral artery
MFB	medial forebrain bundle
MMPI	Minnesota Multiphasic Personality Inventory
MRA	Magnetic Resonance Angiography
MRT	Magnetic Resonance Tomography
NA-SAB	spontaneous non-traumatic SAH without proven source of the bleeding
ns	not significant
PCoA	posterior communicating artery
PET	Positron Emission Tomography

PI	proactive interference
PICA	posterior inferior cerebellar artery
PTSD	post traumatic stress disorder
rCBF	regional cerebral blood flow
rtPA	recombinant plasminogen activator
SAH	subarachnoid hemorrhage
SD	standard deviation
SIADH	secretion inhibition of antidiuretic hormone
SIP	Sickness Impact Profile
SPECT	Single-Photon-Emission-Computed-Tomography
TCD	transcranial Doppler sonography
Triple "H"-Therapy	hypertensive, hypervolemic, hemodynamic therapy
WAIS-R	Wechsler Adult Intelligence Scale-Revised
WCST	Wisconsin Card Sorting Test
WFNS	World Federation of Neurological Surgeons
WHO	World Health Organisation
WIP	short version of the Hamburg-Wechsler Intelligence test
WMS	Wechsler-Memory-Scale

1. Introduction

The first description of intracranial aneurysms dates back to the 17th century (Wiseman, 1676). However, two further centuries went by until Hodgson (1815) and later Bramwell (1886) recognized the extravasation of blood under the arachnoid of the brain as the consequence of the rupture of an intracranial aneurysm and named this form of hemorrhage "subarachnoid hemorrhage" (SAH). Until the beginning of the 20th century, a specific and systematic treatment of ruptured intracranial aneurysms was not possible because of the lack of adequate diagnostics (Beadles, 1907; Keen, 1890). The surgical treatment of ruptured intracranial aneurysms developed very slowly and was, despite all efforts, associated with a considerable mortality and morbidity. However, an enormous progress in neurosurgical treatment methods within the last 30 years has led to a considerable improvement of the prognosis. The introduction of the operating microscope, the concept of early surgery within 72 hours of the bleeding, specialized intensive care units, the calcium antagonist nimodipine and a highly differentiated pre- and post-operative management have contributed essentially to this advance (Hütter et al., 1999; Ljunggren, Sharma and Buchfelder, 1993; Kassell et al., 1990a;b; Gilsbach and Harders, 1989; Gilsbach et al., 1988a; Ljunggren et al., 1987; Drake, 1981). This implies that in the meantime 50–60% of all patients after the rupture of one or more intracranial aneurysms can be regarded as functional survivors (Kassell et al., 1990a;b; Gilsbach and Harders, 1989; Gilsbach et al., 1988a; Ljunggren et al., 1987).

Taking into account that most patients are stricken by SAH in the middle of their lives, the question of the quality of life of the survivors becomes of increasing importance, especially in the face of medical progress (Hütter and Gilsbach, 1996b; 1995b; Hütter, Gilsbach and Kreitschmann, 1995; Vilkki et al., 1990; McKenna et al., 1989a; Ljunggren et al., 1985). Against this background, the interest in the scientific pursuit of the neurobehavioral late sequelae of SAH results from three different motives:

1. Due to the progress in neurosurgical treatment of SAH caused by the rupture of an intracranial aneurysm, a sharp decrease of the mortality and morbidity of this formerly fatal illness could be achieved (Ljunggren, Sharma and Buchfelder, 1993; Kassell et al., 1990a;b; Gilsbach and Harders, 1989; Gilsbach et al., 1988a; Ljunggren et al., 1985; Drake, 1981; Norlen and Olivecrona, 1953). It is, therefore, of considerable interest to ascertain if and to what extent psychosocial impairments exist in the now much increased patient group of functional survivors after SAH.

Moreover, further points of interest concern the causes of these impairments as well as treatment and preventional aspects.
2. The other source of scientific curiosity in the neurobehavioral sequelae of SAH stems from the discipline of neuropsychology, where the cognitive and psychosocial impairments connected to this illness have been a matter of interest for quite some time (Hütter, Gilsbach and Kreitschmann, 1995; Vilkki et al., 1990; Ljunggren et al., 1985; Sengupta, Chin and Brierley, 1975; Penrose and Storey, 1970; Logue et al., 1968; Storey, 1970;1967). This preoccupation may mainly be put down to frequent reports published since the fifties and sporadically even earlier on spectacular neuropsychological disorders such as amnestic syndromes and changes of personality up to pronounced brain organic syndromes in this patient group (Storey, 1970;1967; Norlen and Lindquist, 1964; Webster et al., 1960; Walton, 1953).
3. A further reason for the neuropsychological interest in the sequelae of SAH is probably explained by the association of the observed impairments with lesions of frontobasal and midline structures, whose importance for cognitive and emotional functions has long been a matter of intensive discussion in neuropsychological research (Richardson and DeLong, 1988; Damasio et al., 1985a;b; Stuss and Benson, 1984; Stuss et al., 1982; Norlen and Lindquist, 1964).

In studies about cognitive deficits and quality of life after SAH, a large number of patients complained about a persistent impairment of their cognitive capacity, as well as increased irritability, change of personality, loss of motivation and emotional problems, although their neurological outcome had been rated according to the Glasgow Outcome Scale (GOS; Jennett and Bond, 1967) for the most part as good (GOS = I) (Ogden, Mee and Henning, 1993a; Hütter and Gilsbach, 1993; Vilkki et al., 1990; Bornstein et al., 1987; Stolke et al., 1987; Auer, Gallhofer and Auer, 1985; Ljunggren et al., 1985). A number of studies about the neuropsychological sequelae of the rupture of an aneurysm published so far show that neither the location of the aneurysm, nor focal brain damage seen on cranial computed tomography (CCT), nor the surgical intervention, but the bleeding itself and hemorrhage-associated secondary brain damage must be regarded as the most important causal factors for the neuropsychological sequelae of SAH (Hütter, Kreitschmann-Andermahr and Gilsbach, 1998; Hütter et al., 1998; Hütter and Gilsbach, 1996a; Satzger et al., 1995; Tidswell et al., 1995; Hütter, Gilsbach and Kreitschmann, 1994; Hütter and Gilsbach, 1993; Ogden, Mee and Henning, 1993a; Hütter and Gilsbach, 1992; Oder et al., 1991; Ogden, Levin and Mee, 1990; Vilkki et al., 1990;1989; Sonesson et al., 1989; DeSantis et al., 1989). It is not yet clear, however, which aspects of the ictus itself and what types of secondary brain damage are associated in which way with the neurobehavioral sequelae of SAH. The scientific clarification of these still unresolved questions requires at first an exact definition of the pathophysiological processes that occur in context with SAH and its treatment.

Proceeding from neurosurgical and neuropsychological concepts, it is the aim of the present work to identify the causal factors for the neuropsychological sequelae of SAH and to clarify the significance of neurosurgical treatment methods from an interdisciplinary point of view. Finally, consequences for future neurosurgical treatment as well as psychosocial care and rehabilitation shall be derived from these results. The long-range aim is to minimize or, if possible, to completely avoid the persistent neurobehavioral impairments in this patient group.

2. Clinical appearance, pathology and diagnostics of subarachnoid hemorrhage (SAH)

2.1. Definition, epidemiology and etiology

Spontaneous subarachnoid hemorrhage is a hemorrhage into the subarachnoid space between the arachnoid layer and the cortical surface of the brain. The subarachnoid space comprises essentially the basal cisterns, the interhemispherical fissure and the Sylvian fissure (Yasargil, 1984). The incidence of SAH lies between 0.06 and 0.08/1000 persons/year (Linn et al., 1996). There are considerable regional differences with a particularly high incidence in Finland of 0.21/1000 persons/year (Linn et al., 1996). Women are affected approximately 1.6 times more often than men (Linn et al., 1996). Smoking, arterial hypertension and alcohol ingestion of more than 150 g per week increase the risk to sustain an SAH (Teunissen et al., 1996; Taylor et al., 1995). According to an epidemiological study on the incidence of cerebrovascular disease in the community of Oxford and surroundings, the most common primary manifestation in a time span of four years was cerebrovascular occlusive disease with 81%, followed by intracerebral hemorrhage (10%) and subarachnoid hemorrhage with an incidence of 5%, as well as 5% unclear cases (Bamford et al., 1990). In so far, SAH represents a much more infrequent illness in comparison to cerebrovascular occlusive disease or traumatic brain injury. In Germany alone a total of approximately 150,000 persons per year are affected by traumatic brain injury with a fatal outcome in 30,000 cases (Gilsbach, Mayfrank and Lennartz, 1996). According to reliable evidence from the USA, the incidence rate of traumatic brain injury is approximated to 200/100,000 persons per year (Kraus, 1987).

In the already cited epidemiological study on the incidence of cerebrovascular disease in Oxford and surroundings, the fatality rate within 30 days of disease onset amounted to 10% in cerebrovascular occlusive disease, to 50% in the case of intracerebral hemorrhage and still to 46% in case of SAH (Bamford et al., 1990). Meanwhile, around 80–85% patients survive their first SAH. The overall mortality (disease and treatment mortality), nevertheless, still amounts to circa 50% (Gilsbach, Poeck and Piscol, 1993; Bamford et al., 1990; Kassell et al., 1990a;b). However, this means that still every third to fourth patient who reaches hospital alive succumbs later on to the disease or the consequences of treatment. In the United States, approximately 14,000 patients per year can be regarded as functional survivors of SAH (Kassell et al., 1990a;b). This implies, after all, that in

Table 1. Causes of spontaneous subarachnoid hemorrhage (SAH)

Cause	%
Aneurysm	51
Hypertension/arteriosclerosis	15
Arteriovenous malformation	6
Others/multiple	6
Unknown	22

According to Sahs et al. (1969)

the last ten years 140,000 persons have survived an SAH in the USA. This number cannot be neglected in the face of the assumedly considerable psychosocial sequelae of the illness. A similar incidence rate can be presumed for Central Europe. Also mortality and morbidity should not be different from the American statistics, although it must be noted that the figures may vary substantially with respect to the different hospitals (Kassell et al., 1990a;b).

In approximately 50% of all cases, SAH is the consequence of a ruptured aneurysm along an artery of the circle of Willis (Yasargil, 1984). A further 15–25% of the bleedings remain without a proven source, although the numbers cited in the literature do vary (Linn et al., 1996; Rinkel, van Gijn and Wijdicks, 1993; Sahs et al., 1969). Table 1 gives an overview of the distribution of causes of spontaneous SAH.

Traumatic SAH as the consequence of traumatic brain injury must also be differentiated from spontaneous SAH. Approximately 30% of all moderate and severe traumatic brain injuries are accompanied by traumatic SAH (McCormick, 1985). In some cases, it is difficult to differentiate between traumatic SAH as the consequence of a fall or an accident from spontaneous non-traumatic SAH without a proven source of the bleeding. Accidents or falls can not only be the cause of SAH but also occur relatively often in its wake. Since the different etiological groups are not comparable, in the following, only spontaneous aneurysmal and spontaneous non-traumatic SAH without a proven source of the bleeding are taken into consideration. For this reason, earlier studies in which this differentiation of SAH into etiologically comparable groups was not realized consequently, can only be interpreted with limitations.

2.2. Epidemiology of SAH as a result of the rupture of an aneurysm and of spontaneous SAH without a proven source of the bleeding

Intracranial aneurysms are outpouchings from the wall of intracranial vessels (Gilsbach, Poeck and Piscol, 1993). An aneurysm develops from a congenital weakness of the vessel wall with a missing media muscularis and a thinning of the elastica, before all in the region of branching and ramification of

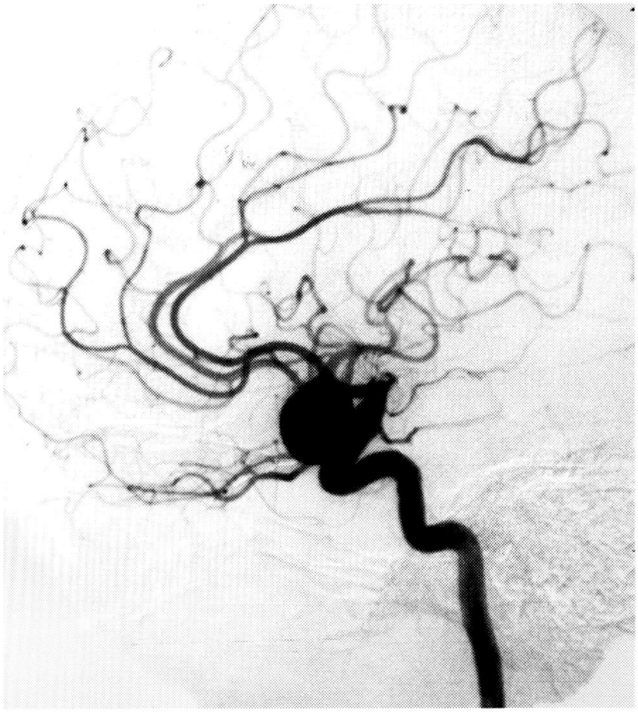

Fig. 1. A supraophthalmic aneurysm of the internal carotid artery

the large intracranial arteries. Figure 1 shows a large supraophthalmic aneurysm of the internal carotid artery.

A typical intracranial aneurysm consists in 90% of all cases of a saccular outpouching from the wall of the cerebral artery, whose point of origin from the parent vessel is referred to as the neck and the curved endpart as the dome or fundus (Gilsbach, Poeck and Piscol, 1993). The range of sizes of intracranial aneurysms reaches from microscopically small outpouchings from the vessel wall and large (diameter > 15 mm) aneurysms up to giant aneurysms with a diameter > 25 mm (Gilsbach, Poeck and Piscol, 1993). The majority of intracranial aneurysms exhibit a diameter between 4 and 15 mm. The rupture of the dilated aneurysmal wall causes a hemorrhage into the subarachnoid space, the subdural space, the cerebral parenchyma and, occasionally, intraventricular hemorrhage. In more than 90%, SAH is the primary manifestation of an aneurysm. Moreover, aneurysms can rarely become symptomatic by compressive effects on neighboring structures or by space-occupying effects in case of special localization or unusual size (giant aneurysms) (Gilsbach, Poeck and Piscol, 1993). Approximately 80–90% of all intracranial aneurysms are located in the anterior part of the circle of Willis, while the remaining 10–20% originate from the vertebro-basilar circulation (Kassell et al., 1990a; Yasargil, 1984). Table 2 gives an overview of the distribution (in percent) of the localization of intracranial aneurysms.

Table 2. Location of surgically treated aneurysms according to their location at the four major intracranial arteries

Vessel/section of vessel	%
Internal carotid a.	32,7
cavernous sinus	0,6
ophthalmic a.	3,4
posterior communicating a.	16,6
anterior choroidal a.	2,5
bifurcation	5,3
others	4,5
Middle cerebral a.	13,0
main trunk	1,7
bifurcation	11,5
Anterior cerebral a.	40,8
anterior communicating a.	35,8
horizontal part	1,4
pericallosal a.	8,4
Basilar/vertebral a.	13,2
bifurcation	6,8
basilar a.	3,9
inferior posterior cerebellar a.	1,7
vertebral a.	0,8
Others	5,0

According to Yasargil (1984) (N = 355)

Intracranial aneurysms (including micro-aneurysms) can be found, according to the results of autopsy studies, in at least 1% (0.2–16%) of the deceased (Taylor et al., 1995; Stehbens, 1963; Hassler, 1961). Of all persons harboring an intracranial aneurysm, one half remain asymptomatic during life, whereas the other half will sustain SAH at some point of time (Taylor et al., 1995; McCormick and Rosenfield, 1973; Graf, 1971). Ten (6–12) aneurysms rupture per 100,000 inhabitants and year (Taylor et al., 1995; Philips et al., 1980; Pakarinen, 1967). The likelihood of an intact aneurysm to rupture lies between 1–2% per year. The incidence is higher in aneurysms with a diameter >5–6 mm, with the majority of ruptured aneurysms exhibiting a diameter of 7 mm and more (Smith and Miller, 1990). Giant aneurysms with a diameter >25 mm have a bleeding rate comparable to small aneurysms (Smith and Miller, 1990). The peak of the age distribution in ruptured aneurysms lies at the age of 50. Aneurysmal SAH at an age below 20 years is rare with a frequency of approximately 2% (Ostergaard and Voldby, 1983; Lipper et al., 1978). On the other hand, some 10% of all patients suffering aneurysmal SAH are more than 60 years of age (Bonita and Thompson, 1985; Yasargil, 1984). Arterial hypertension, arteriosclerosis and lipopathy are discussed as risk factors for the rupture of an aneurysm

(Gilsbach, Poeck and Piscol, 1993). An intracranial aneurysm can rupture without a perceivable cause and take the affected person by surprise during rest or sleep. More often, however, tangible emotional and/or physical strain (lifting, straining, bending, sexual intercourse, stress, strong emotions) gives rise to the ictus (Ogden, Mee and Henning, 1993b; Nyström, 1973). Seasonal and meterological influences on the frequency of rupture are also noted (Tsementzis et al., 1991). Chyatte et al. (1994) found a substantial influence of changes of the global weather condition within 72 hours on the frequency of rupture of intracranial aneurysms. This correlation could only be confirmed in men but not in women (Chyatte et al., 1994).

The role of arterial hypertension in aneurysm formation is a matter of debate (Taylor et al., 1995). Still, it can be regarded as certain that neither hypertension nor arteriosclerosis alone can be considered exclusive causes for the genesis of an aneurysm (Teunissen et al., 1996; Kassell et al., 1990a). For 90% of all aneurysms, congenital or postnatally acquired factors, or a combination of the two, are discussed (Gilsbach, Poeck and Piscol, 1993). In the remaining 10%, infectious-inflammatory, traumatic or typical arterio-sclerotic alterations can be established. Some 15% (6–32%) of the patients harbor more than one aneurysm (Fox, 1983). More than 6–8 aneurysms in one individual patient are a rarity. Approximately one half of multiple aneurysms originate from the internal carotid artery (in part symmetrically bilateral), one third of the middle cerebral artery, 15% of the anterior communicating artery and some 5% of the vertebro-basilar circulation (Yasargil, 1984). It remains to be stated that the new formation of an aneurysm can occur after angiographical exclusion of multiple aneurysms and surgical elimination of an aneurysm in less than 1% of all patients (Marchel, Bidzinski and Bojarski, 1991; Koeleveld et al., 1991).

2.3. Pathophysiology of SAH

Caused by transgression of the endurance limit of an aneurysmatically dilated wall segment of a cerebral vessel, due to pressure and shearing forces, induced by blood pressure fluctuations, pulse waves or blood flow, the sudden rupture of an aneurysm occurs (Kim et al., 1992; Steiger et al., 1988; 1987; Steiger and Reulen, 1986). Blood forces its way in more than 90% of all cases into the subarachnoid space and causes a so-called SAH. Depending on the direction of the blood flow, it may also enter the cerebral parenchyma (intracerebral hemorrhage) or the ventricular system (intra-ventricular hemorrhage), although the latter is more often the result of a secondary breakthrough of an intracerebral hematoma. A bleeding into the subdural space (subdural hematoma) is much less common. The primary symptoms of SAH depend on the severity of the bleeding, the degree and functional relevance of the destroyed brain tissue, the ensuing rise in intracranial pressure and the disruption of cerebral function. The hemor-rhage is terminated by the extravascular rise in pressure as a consequence of the bleeding and/or by tamponade of the vacant surroundings (Brinker,

Seifert and Dietz, 1992; Grote and Hassler, 1988; Nornes, 1978;1973). The risk of recurrent hemorrhage is high. It can occur at any time with an increase in mortality with every recurrent hemorrhage of approximately 30% (Gilsbach, Poeck and Piscol, 1993). The risk of rebleeding is much lower in SAH without an angiographically proven source of the bleeding, which can be approximated to 10% (Ferbert, Hubo and Biniek, 1992; Oder et al., 1991).

In summary, it can be stated that the primary consequences of SAH caused by a ruptured aneurysm consist of an abrupt rise in intracranial pressure with a more or less protracted collapse or impairment of cerebral perfusion (Brinker, Seifert and Dietz, 1992; Grote and Hassler, 1988; Nornes, 1978;1973). Perifocal or diffuse brain edema and impairment of cerebrospinal fluid resorption (in at least 25% of all patients in the acute phase) belong, after the primary pathophysiological aftermaths, to the secondary consequences that may lead to raised intracranial pressure (Hornyak, Gilsbach and Harders, 1991; Vassilouthis and Richardson, 1979). Malresorption of cerebrospinal fluid and brain edema result in an impairment of cerebral perfusion which can be detected by different methods (Mountz et al., 1991; Matsuda, Shiino and Handa, 1990).

2.4. Clinical features of acute SAH

A sudden, severe headache originating from the neck "as never before" or "like a bolt from the blue", also described as a "crushing headache" is typical for the rupture of an aneurysm. Together with meningism which may arise hours later, this sudden devastating headache constitutes the characteristic main symptom of SAH. As the second most common initial symptom, a clouding of consciousness which may reach from slight confusion to deep coma usually supervenes. According to evidence from Gilsbach, Poeck and Piscol (1993), depression of consciousness from somnolence to coma occurs in approximately 40% of all patients. In unconscious patients there is generally no meningism. In 25% of all patients, the headache is accompanied by vegetative symptoms such as nausea and vomiting (Gilsbach, Poeck and Piscol, 1993). Shivering, sweating, reactive hypertension and cardiac arrythmias constitute further vegetative symptoms of SAH. Electrocardiographic abnormalities up to a heart attack-like picture, gastrointestinal or pulmonal pathologies up to acute pulmonal edema can be caused by the release of neurohumoral factors. Neurological deficits, mostly in the sense of cerebral nerve palsies or a hemiparesis can supervene. Other focal deficits such as aphasia are more likely caused by an accompanying intracerebral hematoma.

Within the first week of onset, SAH often leads to hypervolemia and a decrease of erythrocytes (Nelson et al., 1991). Epileptic seizures can occur in patients with unruptured aneurysms as well as pre- and postoperatively. The risk varies according to the literature between 3% and 26% (Rabinowick

Table 3. Symptoms of aneurysmal SAH

Symptoms	%
Meningeal irritation	
earlier warning leaks (headache)	30–50
severe headache	>85
nausea and/or vomiting	>50
meningism (after 12–24 hours)	>70
Neurological/neuropsychological deficits	>30
visual field defects	
oculomotor palsy	
hemiparesis	
aphasia	
disorientation/agitation	
Epileptic seizures	4–26
Clouding of consciousness/coma	>40
Sudden death	>15

According to Fox (1983) and Smith and Miller (1990)

et al., 1991; Sbeigh, Tamas and O'Laoire, 1986). Table 3 sums up the symptoms of aneurysmal SAH and their frequency.

First described by Ecker and Riemenschneider (1951), vasospasm constitutes the most frequent cause of morbidity and mortality in connection with SAH next to the immediate consequences of the bleeding (Pool, 1958). By means of cranial computed tomography (CCT), nuclear magnetic resonance imaging (MRI) as well as investigations that depict regional cerebral blood flow (rCBF) and positron emission tomography (PET), ischemic and infarcted brain regions could be shown in about 20% of all patients after the rupture of an aneurysm (Hasan et al., 1992; Mountz et al., 1991; Matsuda, Shiino and Handa, 1990). Vasospasm of the cerebral vessels, proven angiographically or by means of transcranial Doppler sonography (TCD), occurring in 80% of all patients in the second week after SAH (Gilsbach, Poeck and Piscol, 1993), is assumed the most important causal factor for these perfusion abnormalities. The term vasospasm is in itself misleading since the narrowing of arteries is not the consequence of a contraction, but results of a necrosis of the vessel wall and a thickening of the tunica intima and media (Hughes and Schianchi, 1978). According to the results of TCD and angiographic studies, vasospasm follows a relatively constant time course (Harders and Gilsbach, 1987; Seiler et al., 1986). This means that vasospasm does not occur within the first three days after aneurysm rupture (Koenig et al., 1979). From the fourth day until the beginning of the second week, vasospasm increases to remain stable until the end of the second week and to decrease from the third week after SAH (Handa et al., 1992; Harders and Gilsbach, 1987).

2.5. Diagnostics of acute SAH

Lumbar puncture, first described by Quincke (1872) and confirmed by Wichern (1911) as the most important method to verify SAH, has played an important role to ascertain the diagnosis. According to Gilsbach, Poeck and Piscol (1993), diagnosis of SAH comprises three steps: 1. proof of SAH, 2. proof of the cause of SAH and 3. proof of associated complications such as hydrocephalus, intracerebral hemorrhage, subdural hematoma and vasospasm. When SAH is suspected clinically, a CCT should be performed first. CCT is the method of choice to verify SAH. Only if no scanner is available, or if the CCT scan was negative, lumbar puncture should be performed (Gilsbach, Poeck and Piscol, 1993). Evidence of SAH on CCT is dependent on the interval between the bleeding and the time point of investigation. While subarachnoid blood is visible on CCT in 97% of all patients on the day of the bleeding, it can be detected on day 5 only in 63%, with a decreasing reliability in the following time period (Hornyak, Gilsbach and Harders, 1991; Kassell et al., 1990b).

Extent, anatomical distribution and severity of SAH as well as intracerebral or sub/epidural hematomas can be determined by means of CCT. Moreover, hemorrhage into the ventricular system, localization and extent of infarction, brain edema as well as accompanying disturbances of CSF circulation up to hydrocephalus are also seen on CCT (Hornyak, Gilsbach and Harders, 1991). Occasionally, thrombosed or calcified parts of the aneurysm are conspicious. A CCT performed with contrast agent also serves to exclude other causes of bleeding such as tumors or arterio-venous malformations. The diffuse distribution of blood in the subarachnoid space cannot be identified well by means of magnetic resonance imaging (MRI), but blood vessels and aneurysms of approximately 3 mm or more in size can be visualized (Gilsbach, Poeck and Piscol, 1993). T2-weighted spin echo sequences as well as the more recent procedure of non-invasive MR-angiography (MRA), which is performed without contrast agent, are suitable for this purpose. The diagnostic reliability of both procedures has not yet been fully clarified and is subject to some limitations (Gilsbach, Poeck and Piscol, 1993). The restricted spatial resolution of MRA makes the identification and localization of smaller aneurysms still difficult. In rare cases of proven SAH and missing angiographical verification of an aneurysm, the location of the bleeding may be narrowed down by means of MRI, if a small parenchymal bleeding, not visible on CCT, has occurred. Also, angiographically occult arterio-venous malformations such as cavernomas which may also be causal for an SAH can be demonstrated by means of MRI (Mourier et al., 1991; Matsumura et al., 1990).

Cerebral angiography is essential for the verification of an aneurysm and for the planning of therapy. It must be performed as four vessel angiography in order to assess the individual vascular anatomy, possible multiple aneurysms or accompanying angiomas as completely as possible. In case of multiple aneurysms, it is possible to decide by means of angiographical criteria which aneurysm must have bled. In approximately 20–30% of all angiographies no aneurysm is detected (Rinkel, van Gijn and Wijdicks, 1993; Ferbert, Hubo and Biniek, 1992). In these circumstances, angiography should be repeated, although proof of an aneurysm, especially in the event of an exclusively perimesencephalic bleeding, is only successful in 1% of all cases (Ferbert, Hubo and Biniek, 1992).

Transcranial Doppler sonography (TCD), which has been introduced only in 1982, represents another important diagnostic tool in connection with SAH (Aaslid, Markwalder and Nornes, 1982). TCD is based on the Doppler effect which is due to the frequency shift of a sound wave that occurs when either the transmitter, the receiver or the reflected medium – the red blood cells in case of TCD – move away from or approach one another. The frequency shift is hereby proportional to the velocity of the movement. Therefore, increases in blood flow velocity caused by the narrowing of arteries can be demonstrated by means of TCD. A satisfactory correlation of the vessel diameter and the increase in blood flow velocity measured by TCD exists for the internal carotid artery (ICA) and the middle cerebral artery (MCA). This does not hold true for the anterior cerebral artery (ACA) because of the frequent collateralization from the contralateral hemisphere (Gilsbach, Poeck and Piscol, 1993). TCD represents a diagnostic tool which allows to monitor the development of potential vasospasm in the individual patient atraumatically and repeatedly. This way, antiischemic treatment measures against vasospasm can be brought into use more effectively and already preventively. Also, a correlation between mean blood flow velocity acceleration, measured by TCD, and cognitive activities has been described (Harders, Laborde and Droste, 1992). TCD is not suitable, however, for the direct proof of an aneurysm. Furthermore, it must always be taken into account when using TCD that only blood flow velocities and not vessel diameters are measured. Vessel narrowing as well as dilatation may cause similar changes in blood flow velocity (Gilsbach, Poeck and Piscol, 1993).

2.6. The most common classification systems to assess the state of a patient and the severity of SAH

The systematic assessment of the state of a patient after SAH does not only have substantial consequences for therapeutic management and prognosis, but also enables communication among different research groups, since standardized scales facilitate the comparability between studies. The different classification systems that are used in connection with SAH can be divided into three different groups. In the first group, the overall state of the patient is assessed with special emphasis on the state of consciousness. In the second group, the severity of SAH is evaluated with respect to different criteria. The third group comprises scales which roughly quantify the later neurological and psychosocial outcome after SAH. In all classifications, the evaluation of the severity of the symptoms after SAH is first of all centered upon the state of consciousness of the patient and the presence

Table 4. Classification of the preoperative clinical state according to the grading of Hunt and Hess (1968)

Grade 1	Mild headache and/or neck stiffness
Grade 2	Severe headache and/or pronounced neck stiffness and/or cranial nerve deficits, photophobia
Grade 3	Drowsiness and/or mild disorientation and/or slight pareses and/or dysphasia
Grade 4	Stupor or sopor and/or fair to severe hemiparesis and/or dysphasia
Grade 5	Coma, decerebrate rigidity, acute middle brain syndrome

or lack of certain neurological signs. In this context, the five-step grading scale of Hunt and Hess (1968) has become very popular (Table 4).

This rating requires, according to Hunt and Hess (1968), an upgrading of one step in case of serious general diseases such as hypertension, diabetes, advanced arteriosclerosis, chronic pulmonary disease as well as severe vasospasm and old age. From the beginning until the present day, the Hunt and Hess scale is often used for the indication and timing of aneurysm surgery (Hütter et al., 1999; Spetzger and Gilsbach, 1994; Kassell, 1990a;b; Gilsbach and Harders, 1989; Gilsbach et al., 1988a; Hunt and Hess, 1968). Further commonly used classification systems of the clinical state of patients after SAH include the scale of Botterell et al. (1956) as well as the scale of the World Federation of Neurological Surgeons (WFNS), published in 1988 (WFNS SAH Scale, 1988). Tables 5 and 6 show the Botterell and WFNS scales.

In the advent of computed tomography for the diagnostics of SAH, Fisher, Kistler and Davis (1980) suggested the so-called "Fisher-Scale",

Table 5. Classification of the clinical state of SAH patients

Grade I	Patient presents with clear consciousness
Grade II	Patient is tired/drowsy but has no neurological deficits
Grade III	Patient is tired/drowsy but presents with neurological deficit(s)
Grade IV	Patient presents with severe neurological deficit(s) and clinical deterioration
Grade V	Moribund or nearly moribund patient

According to Botterell et al. (1956)

Table 6. Classification of the clinical state of SAH patients according to the WFNS SAH scale (1988)

Grade	GCS[1]	Motor deficit
I	15	none
II	14–13	none
III	14–13	present
IV	12–7	present or not present
V	6–3	present or not present

[1]GCS = Glasgow Coma Score (Jennett and Teasdale, 1977)

Table 7. Classification of the severity of SAH seen on CCT scan according to the grading system of Fisher, Kistler and Davis (1980)

Grade 0	No blood can be detected on CCT scan
Grade 1	Diffuse distribution or thin, localized layer of blood in all vertical layers (interhemispheric fissure, insular cistern, ambient cistern) less than 1 mm of thickness
Grade 2	Localized clots of blood and/or vertical layers of blood more than 1 mm of thickness
Grade 3	Diffuse or no subarachnoid blood; but intracerebral or intraventricular blood

which rates the severity of SAH according to CCT criteria such as extent, amount and rough anatomical distribution of the bleeding. Table 7 gives an overview of the classification of the severity of SAH on the basis of CCT after the scale of Fisher, Kistler and Davis (1980).

Gilsbach et al. (1988a) used a modified version of the Fisher CCT grading scheme. Table 8 shows the modified Fisher CCT scheme as applied in numerous studies of the research group around Gilsbach.

For the more differentiated evaluation of the severity of SAH on the basis of CCT findings, Hijdra et al. (1990) suggested an assessment scale based on the evaluation and summation of the quantity of blood in 10 of the individual subarachnoid compartments listed in Fig. 2. The amount of blood is determined by means of the following semiquantitative scale: 0 = no blood; 1 = small quantity of blood; 2 = moderate quantity of blood; 3 = completely filled with blood. The SAH sum score as the expression of the total amount of subarachnoid blood is calculated by addition of the quantities of blood determined for the ten individual subarachnoid compartments. This means that the SAH sum score according to the assessment scheme of Hijdra et al. (1990) can take on values between 0 and 30.

Le Roux proposed a rating scheme, initially developed for the assessment of the amount of intraventricular blood after traumatic brain injury (Le Roux et al., 1992). This rating is also suitable for the quantification of intraventricular blood after hemorrhages of other etiology (Mayfrank, 1997; Mayfrank et al., 1997a). Table 9 gives an overview of the evaluation criteria for the severity of intraventricular hemorrhage (IVH) from which an IVH-

Table 8. Modified Fisher CCT grading system for quantification of the severity of SAH

Grade 0	No blood present: no blood can be detected on CCT scan
Grade 1	Mild: thin, localized layer of blood
Grade 2	Moderate: thick layers of blood in two of three subarachnoid compartments or in one and on the cortical surface
Grade 3	Severe: extended, diffuse SAH with thick layers of blood in all subarachnoid compartments or in two and on the cortical surface Intracerebral hematoma > 2 cm

According to Gilsbach et al. (1988a)

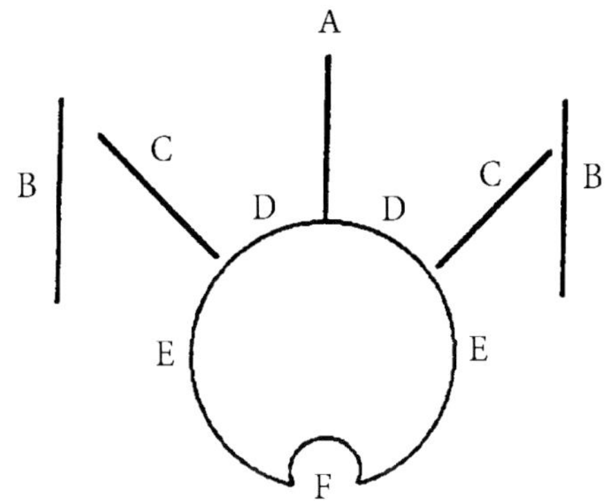

Fig. 2. Calculation of the SAH sum score according to Hijdra et al. (1990). Schematic representation of the ten basal cisterns and fissures (*A–F*), used for the evaluation of the quantity of blood: *A* frontal interhemispheric fissure; *B* lateral part of the Sylvian fissure; *C* proximal (medio-basal) part of the Sylvian fissure; *D* suprasellar cistern; E ambient cistern; *F* quadrigeminal cistern (according to Hijdra et al., 1990)

Table 9. Criteria for the assessment of the severity of IVH

Score	Description
1	Small sedimentation of blood
2	Less than half of one ventricle is filled with blood
3	More than half of one ventricle is filled with blood
4	The whole ventricle is filled with blood and dilated

According to Le Roux et al. (1992)

score as an expression of the severity of the entire intraventricular hemorrhage can be calculated (Le Roux et al., 1992).

The IVH-score is calculated by addition of the scores of the four individual ventricles, the maximal IVH-score is, therefore, 16 (Le Roux et al., 1992).

For the evaluation of the overall outcome after SAH, the Glasgow Outcome Scale (GOS), published in 1967 by Jennett and Bond for the quantification of treatment outcome of patients after traumatic brain injury, is frequently used (Jennett and Bond, 1967). The GOS was developed by the authors for the purpose of facilitating communication between research groups by means of operationalized outcome criteria and to advance the development of prognosis models of treatment outcome (Jennett and Bond, 1967). In order to enable a simple and reliable assessment, Jennett and Bond (1967) deliberately restricted themselves in the conceptualization of the GOS to the physical functional level of the patients. The GOS is composed of three categories of conscious survival and two further categories (Jennett and Bond, 1967). Table 10 gives a survey of the five steps of the GOS and the definition of the categories.

Table 10. The Glasgow Outcome Scale (GOS)

Result	Definition
GOS I	no/minimal impairment
GOS II	modest impairment (needs no help for daily life)
GOS III	severely impaired (needs help for daily life)
GOS IV	persistent vegetative state
GOS V	patient is dead

According to Jennett and Bond (1967)

Initially, the classification of results of the GOS had been laid down by Jennett and Bond (1967) in the opposite manner, with the steps ranging from GOS = I "patient is dead" to GOS = V "minimal or no impairment". In the more recent scientific literature, the reverse scoring, presented in the table above, has become generally accepted.

Much less frequently than the GOS, the Barthel Index (BI) is used to quantify the functional outcome after SAH (Carter et al., 1996). The BI had initially been developed to quantify the capacities in everyday life of patients after stroke (Mahoney and Barthel, 1965), but is used, presently, also in other neurological illnesses. The BI covers 10 functions of everyday life, which are scored by a different number of points, depending on whether they can be accomplished not at all, with help or alone. The possible number of points can vary between 0 and 100 points, with a score of 100 points indicating a far-reaching independency and lack of complaints (Mahoney and Barthel, 1965). Table 11 gives an overview of the items of the Barthel Index and their scoring.

In order to also assess further generally important aspects of daily life, social impairments and the aphasias which are common after stroke, Huber

Table 11. The Barthel Index

Function	With help points	Autonomous points
1. Eating	5	10
2. Change from bed to wheel chair	5–10	15
3. Personal hygiene	0	5
4. Use of toilet	5	10
5. Use of washroom	0	5
6. Ability to walk 50 m on even ground (also with a stick)	10	15
7. Ability to mount stairs (with assistance)	5	10
8. Getting dressed (without shoes)	5	10
9. Control of faeces	5	10
10. Control of bladder	5	10

According to Mahoney and Barthel (1965)

et al. (1990) extended the initial BI by ten items. These additional items refer to 1. orientation to time, place and person, 2. memory, 3. insight into linguistic inconsistencies, 4. the capability of verbal expression, 5. the capability to answer questions correctly with 'yes' or 'no', 6. the ability to prepare simple meals, 7. the participation in family events, 8. the ability to undertake walks or excursions, 9. the ability to master normal shopping for groceries, and, 10. the ability to participate in cultural, religious or social events (Huber et al., 1990).

2.7. Natural course of SAH

After a mild SAH, the patient recovers, when vasospasm does not occur, spontaneously within days. After more severe hemorrhages, the life-threatening state persists over a longer period of time and abates only gradually. A deterioration of the clinical state up to death is possible at any time. In approximately 15–40% of all patients, the initial bleeding is so severe, that they do not reach hospital alive or die soon after admission (Ljunggren et al., 1988;1987; Fox, 1983). Those patients who survive their first SAH are endangered by three major complications: 25–30% do not recover from the immediate consequences of the bleeding, of those who get better, 25–50% deteriorate again from a rebleeding within the following two weeks, and a further 11–34% sustain lethal or disabling delayed ischemic neurological deficits due to cerebral vasospasm (Gallhofer and Auer, 1982; Gilsbach et al., 1990).

Rebleeding, vasospasm, brain edema, secondary IVH, acute hydrocephalus and metabolic disturbances are the main complications of the spontaneous course (Gilsbach, Poeck and Piscol, 1993). Without surgical treatment of the aneurysm, a rebleeding with an increased mortality of 45% (30–70%) occurs in about 40% (25–50%) of all patients (Gallhofer and Auer, 1982). The first hours and days after the initial hemorrhage can be regarded as particularly critical (Inagawa, 1994). There is no peak time for rebleeding within this time span. Rather, the risk decreases day by day (Jane et al., 1985; Kassell and Torner, 1983). It is the rule, however, that the risk of rebleeding increases with a larger size of the aneurysm and the severity of the initial hemorrhage. After six months, the danger of a lethal rebleeding amounts to 1–2% per year. Lethal rebleedings are possible after several years, even decades after the initial SAH, with a particularly high risk in case of large and giant aneurysms (Hashimoto and Handa, 1982). Clinically manifest vasospasm occurs in 15–60% of all patients (Gilsbach, Poeck and Piscol, 1993). In the past, fatalities and persisting deficits were frequent in this case, however, the number has sunk to 5–11% due to modern treatment strategies (Gilsbach, Poeck and Piscol, 1993). The overall prognosis of the spontaneous course after survival of the initial hemorrhage is poor. In the literature, mortality rates of 25% within the first week, 50% within two months and 70% within 5 years are reported (Winn et al., 1983; Nibbelink, Torner and Henderson, 1977; Graf, 1971).

3. Therapy of SAH

3.1. General principles

In case of SAH due to an acutely ruptured intracranial aneurysm, there are two therapeutic goals: First, to prevent a rebleeding, and, secondly, to treat and to prevent the primary and secondary complications of the bleeding (Gilsbach, Poeck and Piscol, 1993). In case of SAH without a proven source of the bleeding, the emphasis is put on the renewed attempt to identify the source of the bleeding as well as on the treatment of the primary and secondary consequences of the bleeding. The time course is in many ways essential in aneurysmal SAH and determines therapeutic decisions. Maintenance of vital functions and vegetative stabilization of the patient is essential in the first few hours after SAH. In this phase, especially after severe bleedings, respiratory dysregulation and hypertensive crises, as the consequence of vegetative dysregulation, are particularly critical. Only in case of space-occupying hematomas with a rapidly progressive clouding of consciousness, an acute surgical removal of the hematoma is indicated. In approximately 25% of all patients, hydrocephalus with an additional impairment of cerebral perfusion caused by a blockade of the subarachnoid space due to the hemorrhage or blood clots, occurs within hours. In this case, an external ventriculostomy is required to lessen the intracranial pressure. Those cases are critical in which an increase of brain volume caused by the bleeding impedes the dilatation of the ventricles. Nevertheless, in this case a disturbance of CSF circulation with a substantial increase of intracranial pressure exists (Bailes et al., 1990). The concept of early aneurysm surgery (within 72 hours after the ictus) that has evolved within the last 20 years implies that angiography must be carried out as early as possible. The surgical clipping of an aneurysm means the exclusion of rerupture with a certainty of about 98%. Beside the operative clipping of an aneurysm, in the last years endovascular forms of therapy aiming to obstruct the aneurysmal lumen with so-called "coils" with the intent to provoke secondary thrombosis of the aneurysm have become of increasing interest (Guglielmi et al., 1991; Hodes et al., 1991). Next to the fact that these therapies are still in the experimental stage and cannot be applied in clinical routine to all cases, some studies demonstrate that this form of therapy may be problematical and that a permanent elimination of the aneurysm by means of endovascular procedures remains questionable (Reul et al., 1997; Spetzger et al., 1996). Coil embolisation has the advantage that the patient is spared the intracranial surgical intervention. The procedure bears, however, its own risks.

These consist in the mechanical damage of the intima of cerebral vessels, a perforation of the aneurysm with acute SAH, the distal occlusion of cerebral vessels followed by cerebral infarction due to washed out coils or thrombuses (Spetzger et al., 1997). According to a literature survey by Spetzger, Rohde and Gilsbach (1997), the rate of therapy-induced mortality in endovascular procedures is approximately as high as in the surgical clipping of the aneurysm. However, these comparisons are restricted first of all by the fact that so far no controlled prospective study on treatment results with a randomized assignment of patients to the treatment groups has been performed. A further problem connected to endovascular procedures is that although the aneurysm is treated, the hemorrhage itself is not. Several neuropsychological studies were able to show, however, that the bleeding itself and associated events have an important influence on the cognitive impairments of patients after SAH (Hütter et al., 1999; Hütter, Kreitschmann-Andermahr and Gilsbach, 1998; Hütter, Gilsbach and Kreitschmann, 1995; 1994; Sonesson et al., 1989).

Since vasospasm is dependent on the quantity of subarachnoid blood, every reduction of the amount of blood in the subarachnoid space can be regarded as a preventive measure against vasospasm or at least as a means to lessen their severity (Adams et al., 1987). The operative removal of the blood within the first two days, at best within the first 24 hours, is advantageous for several reasons. First, within the first 24 hours the blood is of a more liquid consistency and can be removed more easily within that time span, while it passes over after two days to a more solid state. Furthermore, an exposition time of at least 48 hours is required for the development of vasospasm, so that the removal of blood on time can prevent vasospasm. Moreover, the overall conditions for the surgical intervention become worse from the second to the third day, because the brain increases in volume due to the development of cerebral edema and then, the blood clots can hardly be removed (Gilsbach, Poeck and Piscol, 1993). In addition, the toxic exposure of the blood or its breakdown products on the vessel walls, probably mediated by oxyhemoglobin, has already taken place (Hughes and Oppenheimer, 1969).

The indication for early surgery (within 72 hours) is usually given in patients in a stadium I–III according to Hunt and Hess, while the indication for surgery in patients in stadium IV–V after Hunt and Hess must be decided upon individually by the neurosurgeon in charge of treatment (Nowak, Schwachenwald and Arnold, 1994; Spetzger and Gilsbach, 1994; Gilsbach, Poeck and Piscol, 1993). Calcium antagonists oftentimes serve as the basic pharmacological treatment for the prevention of delayed ischemic neurological deficits. Especially for nimodipine, an antiischemic effect could be shown in many – also in controlled – studies (Öhman, Servo and Heiskanen, 1991a;b; Gilsbach et al., 1990; Gilsbach, 1988; Öhman and Heiskanen, 1988; Reulen and Philippon, 1988). Induced hypertensive and hypervolemic hemodynamic therapy has proven to be effective in symptomatic vasospasm as well as under preventional aspects. This hypertensive, hypervolemic hemodilution (Triple "H"-Therapy) is based on the principle to induce mild to more pronounced hypervolemia and hemodilution in the patient using electrolyte solutions, plasma derivatives or dextrane solutions and to elevate systolic blood pressure artificially by the catecholamines dopamine, dobutamine, adrenaline, and/or noradrenaline (Kreitschmann-Andermahr and Gilsbach, 1996; Kreitschmann-Andermahr, Hütter and Gilsbach, 1996; 1995; Bailes et al., 1990; Origitano et al., 1990; Awad et al., 1987). A further, more controversial treatment alternative includes the superselective intraarterial infusion of papaverine (Kaku et al., 1992). The early and appropriate operative elimination of the aneurysm and a consequent postoperative management based on nimodipine and Triple"H"-Therapy, initiated already in case of beginning vasospasm reduces lethal outcomes or permanent impairments due to vasospasm to 2% (Gilsbach and Harders, 1989).

An early surgical removal of blood clots in combination with a postoperative external cisternal drain would also appear suitable for the treatment of the secondary consequences of SAH. The surgical results indicate, indeed, a lower incidence of vasospasm (Inagawa, Kamiya and Matsuda, 1991; Inagawa, Yamamoto and Kamiya, 1990). However, the bilateral trepanation required in this case did nor gain general acceptance. Most recently, pharmacological treatment options evolved that bring about a lysis of the coagulated blood in the subarachnoid space using recombinant tissue plasminogen activator (rtPA) (Mayfrank, 1997; Mayfrank et al., 1997a;b; Schaller, Rohde and Hassler, 1995; Mayfrank et al., 1993; Findlay, Grace and Weir, 1993; Stolke and Seifert, 1992; Findlay et al., 1991; 1990; Seifert et al., 1989b), after prior attempts with streptokinase and urokinase did not prove to be successful. The substance rtPA, produced by means of gene technology, acts fibrigenolytic only in the extravascular compartment, so that the bleeding risk remains small. Yet, the subarachnoid blood can dissolve and drain off via a catheter (Mayfrank et al., 1997a;b; Stolke and Seifert, 1992; Findlay et al., 1991; 1990).

3.2. Operative therapy of ruptured intracranial aneurysms

3.2.1. The historical development of aneurysm surgery

The specific operative treatment of intracranial aneurysms only became possible with the development of cerebral angiography by Moniz (1927), as the fundamental prerequisite for the proof and localization of the cerebral aneurysm. Before the development of suitable removable aneurysm clips at the end of the nineteen seventies, the so-called "trapping", during which the aneurysm-bearing vessel was eliminated, was a common surgical procedure. This led, however, to frequent ischemic complications. An interesting historic study on this matter, dealing with the psychological sequelae of the unilateral occlusion of the anterior cerebral artery (ACA) has been performed by Webster et al. (1960). In 50 patients with occlusion of the proximal ACA, proven by angiography, the authors noted an overall impairment of intellectual fuctions, reduced introspection, anxiety attacks, loss of incentive and impaired reasoning abilities, next to neurological symptoms. The neuropsychological symptoms also occurred when no neurological deficit was present (Webster et al., 1960). Another historic surgical treatment method was to wrap the aneurysm with muscle tissue, also called "coating". This procedure, too, did not prove to be a success (Ogilvy and Poletti, 1991). The thus treated aneurysms had, as well as incompletely clipped ones, a high rate of re-rupture (Feuerberg et al., 1987; Drake, Friedman and Peerless, 1984; Drake and Vanderlinden, 1967).

Beadles (1907) reported that already in 1885 Sir Victor Horsley attempted to eliminate intracranial aneurysms by means of ligature of the internal carotid artery (ICA). During one operation, he retracted both frontal lobes to discover an aneurysm of the skull base, that compressed the optic chiasm and produced visual disturbances. Horsley used the ligature of both internal carotid arteries. The patient survived the intervention and only died several years later. A further patient was operated upon by Beadles who occluded the right ICA by means of ligature. Five years after surgery the patient is said to have been of excellent health (Beadles, 1907). The first report on a premature intraoperative rupture of an aneurysm comes from the Norwegian surgeon Vilhelm Magnus, who incidentally discovered a giant intracavernous aneurysm of the ICA in 1924 when exploring the middle fossa of a patient suffering of trigeminal neuralgia. The aneurysm ruptured and caused a massive hemorrhage. After all, the bleeding could be stopped and the patient survived with severe, permanent impairments (Magnus, 1927). A historic report on a successful aneurysm elimination stems from Nattrass (1928), who gave the account of how Grey Turner in 1926 occluded a suspected aneurysm of the ICA in the cavernous sinus in a patient approximately 12 weeks after SAH by means of ligature. At follow-up one year later, the patient had recovered fully except for diplopia and also the psychopathological disturbances, present before surgery, had returned to normal (Nattrass, 1928).

Walter Dandy first operated an intracranial aneurysm in 1928 (Albright, 1929). The patient bore an aneurysm of the ICA/PCoA (posterior communicating artery) which had caused a palsy of the third cranial nerve. In this patient Dandy had used the ligature of the ICA as customary at the time, however, the patient died a few days later due to massive cerebral infarction (Albright, 1929). According to Ljunggren, Sharma and Buchfelder (1993) Norman Dott is supposed to have completed the first successful early surgery for an intracranial aneurysm on April 22, 1931. Dott operated a patient two days after his third SAH within two weeks on an aneurysm of the middle cerebral artery (MCA), which he wrapped with muscle tissue. Already a few days after surgery the patient was responsive again and recovered so far within the following two years, that he was able to pursue his old hobbies. Without any sign of a further hemorrhage, he died 11 years after this operation of heart disease (Ljunggren, Sharma and Buchfelder,

1993). Dott used the wrapping procedure again in 1931 and 1932 in two further patients, both bearing large aneurysms. However, the first patient died within 24 hours of the intervention of a rebleeding, whereas the other died five days later due to pneumonia (Ljunggren, Sharma and Buchfelder, 1993). In a young nurse, Dott performed an acute operation again in 1932. Four days after repeated SAH, he treated an aneurysm by means of ligature of the ICA. The patient recovered so far, that she was able to take up her old profession as a nurse again. (Ljunggren, Sharma and Buchfelder, 1993). Dott (1933) also gave an account of the successful surgical treatment of ruptured aneurysms of the left ICA. The surgical techniques used by Dott (1933) were the wrapping of the aneurysm and, in other cases, the ligature of the ICA proximally to the site of rupture. All four patients recovered completely from their left-sided oculomotor palsy, and, in two patients, according to Dott (1933), aphasia was reversible (Dott, 1933). Between 1932 and 1936, Dott carried out a total of eight surgical procedures in which he treated aneurysms by means of ligature of the ICA. Of the eight patients, five attained an overall good neurological result (Dott, 1969).

Walter Dandy reported in 1938 of an operation, carried out by himself in 1936, where he had been able to eliminate an aneurysm of the right ICA using the "trapping" procedure (Dandy, 1938). Unfortunately, Dandy (1938) does not give account of eventual neuropsychological or psychopathological disturbances in the patient. Only one year later, Dandy (1939) reported the first successful use of a clip for aneurysm surgery. Dandy eliminated the ICA aneurysm surgically by placing a McKenzie silver clip across the neck of an aneurysm near the origin of the PCoA (Dandy 1939). As to the surgical treatment of aneurysms of the MCA and anterior communicating artery (ACoA), Dandy (1944) was very reserved because of his experiences. All four patients operated upon by him on an MCA aneurysm had died postoperatively of the consequences of surgery (Dandy, 1944). Schorstein (1944) provided an overview of all cases available at the time in whom non-traumatic saccular intracranial aneurysms had been treated by means of ligature of the ICA. Of the 60 cases collected by Schorstein, 8 (13%) had died of the consequences of the operation and 8 (13%) had sustained a hemiplegia (Schorstein, 1944).

3.2.2. Technical improvements in aneurysm surgery

An extremely important date for the treatment of cerebral aneurysm is July 1932, when Moniz and Lima first succeeded in demonstrating an intracranial aneurysm by means of angiography (Ljunggren, Sharma and Buchfelder, 1993). A second milestone was the introduction of removable clips. Not satisfactorily placed clips could be removed and repositioned. Moreover, temporary clipping of vessels became possible. In the nineteen fifties, Olivecrona developed an especially long removable clip for the occlusion of an aneurysm. Further technical improvements followed with the clips by

Schwartz and Mayfield and the particularly light-weight, curved clips by Scoville, introduced in the sixties (Ljunggren, Sharma and Buchfelder, 1993).

In the 1960s and early 1970s, further technical improvements in neurosurgery arose with the development of cranial computed tomography (CCT) and the first steps toward the introduction of the operating microscope, ushering in a quantum leap for the treatment of ruptured intracranial aneurysms. In the early sixties, Thoralf Sundt procured a microscope for the neurosurgical laboratory at the Mayo Clinic, as he was convinced of its usefulness for aneurysm surgery. Already in 1964, Adams and Witt were the first to report of the use of the operating microscope during surgery for intracranial aneurysms (Adams and Witt, 1964). Further technical developments and adjustments of the operating microscope to neurosurgical requirements, such as the introduction of an observer tube for the assistent or the addition of especially adapted illumination, ensued in the following years. The birthplace of cerebrovascular microsurgery, however, lies in Vermont at the local university hospital, where Gazi Yasargil carried out a number of experimental studies on cerebrovascular surgery under the microscope which he extended until the routine use of the operating microscope at the University Hospital of Zurich where he became head of the neurosurgical department. The other important development for neurosurgery and especially for the treatment of ruptured intracranial aneurysms consisted of the invention of the first computed tomograph by Hounsfield (Hounsfield, 1973). Already in 1971 the first suitable CCT-scanner for clinical application which had been constructed exclusively for cerebral imaging, was installed in London at Wimbledon Hospital.

Already in 1958, a group of neurosurgeons in the British town of Manchester propagated the concept of early surgery for the definite elimination of the aneurysm and for the removal of blood from the subarachnoid space, in order to prevent the feared ischemic complications (Johnson, Potter and Reid, 1958). Still in the same year, also Pool pleaded for early surgery of ruptured intracranial aneurysms in order to obviate the, in his opinion, dangerous re-ruptures and vasospasms (Pool, 1958). Also Hunt, Meagher and Barnes concurred with Pool's position in 1960 (Hunt, Meagher and Barnes, 1960). In 1965, Norlen adopted the view that those patients in a good initial neurological state should be operated upon early on the first or second day after the bleeding, since the high mortality of re-rupture would justify an active surgical standpoint (Norlen, 1965).

However, only with the introduction of the operating microscope supported by the increasing propagation of the CCT, the technical prerequisites for the re-introduction of the concept of early surgery of ruptured cerebral aneurysms beginning in the 1970s could be established (Hori and Suzuki, 1979; Sano and Saito, 1978; Suzuki, Yoshimoto and Onuma, 1978; Suzuki and Yoshimoto, 1973). Norlen reported results in 1975 of 45 patients operated upon within the first week after aneurysm rupture of whom only 4% had died (Norlen, 1975). Only one year later (1976) at the conference of the American Association of Neurosurgeons (AANS) in San

Francisco, Suzuki and Sano reported their encouraging personal experiences with early surgery of intracranial aneurysms. The extended series of these early operated patients was published by Suzuki, Onuma and Yoshimoto in 1979.

Such results were regarded quite doubtfully for a long time because of the common opinion that early surgery, because it was regarded as more difficult technically, meant an unwarranted risk for the patient and should, therefore, be refused. In summary, it can be stated that at the end of the seventies, the early operative treatment of ruptured aneurysms was propagated increasingly coming from Japan and Scandinavia in order to lower the rate of re-rupture and vasospasm (Mizukami et al., 1982; Suzuki, Onuma and Yoshimoto, 1979; Sano and Saito, 1978; Norlen, 1975). Also in Germany, the concept of early surgery only became accepted hesitatingly. When Eggert and Gilsbach in 1980 reported their first results on early aneurysm surgery at a meeting of the research group for microneurosurgery in Bremen (Gilsbach and Eggert, 1983), surgical exclusion of the aneurysm in the first days after the bleeding was regarded as too dangerous and refused by many neurosurgeons.

3.2.3. Modern surgical treatment of ruptured intracranial aneurysms

Modern surgical therapy of cerebral aneurysms consists essentially in the principle of identifying the aneurysm-bearing vessel after directed trephination and to exclude the aneurysm from circulation by placing a clip across its neck. Figure 1 shows the chronological time course from the rupture of the aneurysm over surgical preparation and clipping until the definite elimination of the aneurysm by bipolar coagulation, using the example of an ACoA aneurysm. It is of particular importance in this case to take notice of the perforating arteries originating from the ACoA, which should – as shown in this figure – be spared under all circumstances.

Surgical clipping is possible in approximately 90% of all cerebral aneurysms with a low mortality and morbidity (Gilsbach, Poeck and Piscol, 1993). Surgical mortality and morbidity depends on the location and difficulty of the aneurysm and lies below 5% for experienced surgeons (Deruty et al., 1992; Yasargil, 1984; Sundt et al., 1982). In giant aneurysms, the surgical difficulty is much higher and, therefore, the frequency of operative mortality and severe neurological impairments can reach up to 30% (Hamburger, Schönberger and Lange, 1992; Drake, 1979; Sundt and Piepgras, 1979). Of the patient characteristics, the preoperative clinical state (Hunt and Hess), accompanying intracerebral hematomas and severe general diseases are most decisive for the operative result (Niskanen et al., 1993; Gerber et al., 1993). The surgical outcome in case of a bad preoperative state (Hunt and Hess grade IV–V) with a satisfactory or good clinical state postoperatively of about 50% is unproportionally worse than in patients in a preoperative state grade I-III after Hunt and Hess, where 80% reach a good or satisfactory postoperative result (Kassell et al., 1990a;b; Gilsbach and

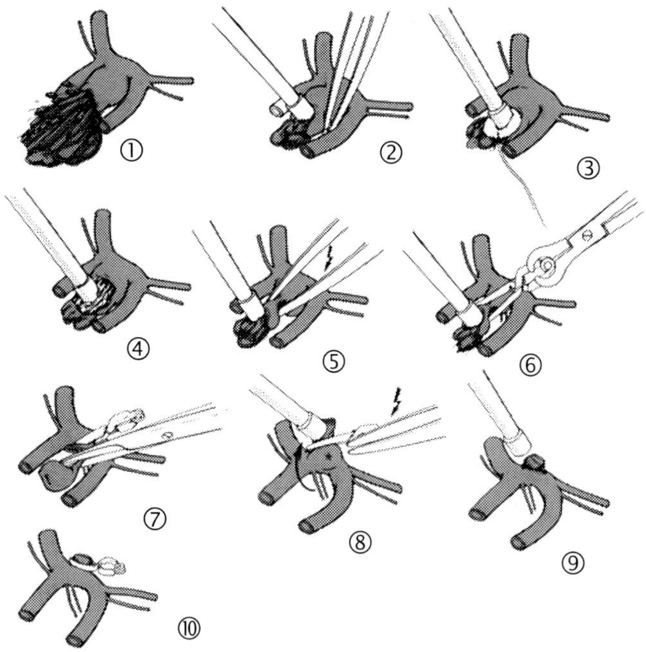

Fig. 1. Surgical treatment of an ACoA aneurysm according to Yasargil (1984)

Harders, 1989; Disney, Weir and Grace, 1988; Gilsbach et al., 1988a). Surgical mortality and morbidity in patients older than 60 years is similar to younger ones (Gilsbach et al., 1988b). Major reasons for surgical impairment of a patient can be found in the inadvertent or inavoidable occlusion of parent or perforating arteries, brain lesions, and massive hemorrhages caused by premature aneurysm rupture before the neck of the aneurysm is exposed well enough to allow clipping (Greenberg, 1984). The risk associated with temporary clipping, that is the temporary occlusion of perforating arteries, is strongly debated (Hütter and Gilsbach, 1996a; Samson et al., 1994; Charbel et al., 1991; Friedmann et al., 1991; Ogawa et al., 1991; Schramm et al., 1990; Wassmann, Werner and Stockert, 1989; Kidooka et al., 1987; Momma, Wang and Symon, 1987; Mooig, Buchthal and Belopavlovic, 1987; Ljunggren et al., 1983). If it is possible at all to speak of a "safe" temporary clipping time of perforating arteries, it is probably shorter than six minutes (Charbel et al., 1992; Friedmann et al., 1991; Ogawa et al., 1991).

The effect of the timing of surgery has been a matter of extensive controversy since the re-introduction of early surgery in the seventies (Hori and Suzuki, 1979; Sano and Saito, 1978, Suzuki and Yoshimoto, 1973), because the accepted general opinion was that intraoperative conditions were much more unfavorable in early surgery than after the consequences of the hemorrhage had worn off. The International Cooperative Study on the Timing of Aneurysm Surgery (Kassell et al., 1990a;b) did not demonstrate any major difference in management mortality and morbidity depending on the timing of surgery. The few comparable studies on early and late surgery showed a better treatment result in favor of early surgery (Chyatte, Fode and Sundt, 1988; Milhorat and Krautheim, 1986; Kassell et al., 1981). Also, according to the results of Gilsbach et al. (1988a), the operative results of early aneurysm surgery in comparison to historical data led to the conclusion that inspite of the perhaps worse technical conditions, early surgery does not have a higher operative mortality and morbidity than late surgery. Provided the appropriate exclusion of the aneurysm by an experienced surgeon, intraoperative aneurysm rupture, inadvertent injury to parent or perforating vessels, direct brain injury and "complicated" surgery are as frequent and followed by the same morbidity and mortality as in late surgery (Hernesniemi et al., 1993; Gilsbach et al., 1990; Gilsbach and Harders, 1989; Gilsbach et al., 1988a;b; Ljunggren et al., 1987; Gilsbach and Eggert, 1983).

The preferred operative approaches for aneurysms of the MCA and ICA are usually fronto-temporal, so-called pterional approaches (Yasargil, 1984). For aneurysms of ACoA interhemispheric as well as pterional approaches are used (Weir, 1993). Aneurysms of the pericallosal artery are approached interhemispherically by means of a frontal unilateral trephination (Ellenbogen and Scott, 1991). The pterional as well as the subtemporal approach is suitable to attack aneurysms of the basilar bifurcation (Babif), the superior cerebellar artery as well as the P1 segment of the posterior cerebral artery (PCA). Several approaches have been suggested for the rare aneurysms of the middle segment of the basilar artery and the anterior inferior cerebellar artery (AICA) to expose this poorly accessible region, reaching from subtemporal, anterosigmoidal to supracondylar and transoral approaches (Pritz, 1991; Drake et al., 1981;1979). Medial unilateral or paracondylar approaches have been developed for aneurysms of the posterior inferior cerebellar artery (PICA) (Bertalanffy and Seeger, 1991).

3.3. Postoperative mortality after aneurysm rupture

Still at the beginning of the 1950s, the treatment mortality in a series of 278 patients after SAH due to the rupture of an intracranial aneurysm amounted to 28%, whereas in smaller series the mortality rates ranged between 8 and 86% (Sahs et al., 1969). In a Scandinavian study based on a series of 138 patients and published in 1950, the authors concluded that 60% of all patients after SAH die sooner or later, whereas 20% survive permanently disabled and only 20% attain an acceptable clinical outcome (Ask-Upmark and Ingvar, 1950). Even in 1957, upon presenting a conference paper, John Holms termed SAH as the most frequent and fastest lethal neurological emergency (Holms, 1958). The most important causes of mortality of surgically treated patients after aneurysm rupture have changed considerably within the last three decades. Macrosurgical approaches, "trapping" of the aneurysm-bearing vessel, and the use of irremovable clips have contributed considerably to fatal outcomes in the sixties. In this decade, the postoperative mortality ranged between 28 and 53% (Troupp and Björksten, 1981; McKissock, Paine and Walshe, 1960).

The postoperative mortality could be lowered dramatically in the nineteen seventies due to the introduction of the operating microscope and technical advancements of the used clips and instruments. The strategy to delay surgery until a time point between the 11th and 14th day after SAH facilitated the intervention technically. Thus, postoperative mortalities between 0 and 2.7% were reported (Milhorat and Krautheim, 1986; Sano and Saito, 1978). The concept of early surgery within 72 hours after SAH was re-introduced for patients after SAH in a good neurological state at the end of the seventies, after the re-rupture of the aneurysm during the time of waiting for surgery had been identified as the most important causal factor for severe impairment or death (Milhorat and Krautheim, 1986; Sundt and Whisnant, 1978). In a series of Milhorat and Krautheim (1986), 65 of 100 patients with aneurysmal SAH thus died during the time of waiting for scheduled late surgery due to re-rupture, vasospasm, and systemic complications. In the 1980s, cerebral vasospasm took the place of re-rupture of the aneurysm as the most important cause of death. This again led to the introduction of active hemodynamic therapy such as triple "H"-therapy and to the development of pharmacological substances like the calcium antagonist nimodipine for the prevention and treatment of cerebral vasospasm (Barker and Ogilvy, 1996; Findlay et al., 1991; Gilsbach et al., 1990; Kassell et al., 1985).

In the years between 1989 and 1997, 390 patients (134 men, 256 women with an age ranging between 16 and 80 years) were operated upon microneurosurgically on an intracranial aneurysm at the Department of Neurosurgery, University Hospital of the University of Technology (RWTH) Aachen. In all patients a modern neurosurgical management consisting of microneurosurgical techniques, the principle of early surgery, a specialized intensive care unit, the use of the calcium antagonist nimodipine and induced hypertension or modified triple "H"-therapy was applied (Kreitschmann-Andermahr and Gilsbach, 1996). 96 (24.6%) of the 390 patients were in a poor neurological state on admission (Hunt and Hess Grad IV order V). In all patients in a clinical state grade I–III according to Hunt and Hess, who had been admitted to the Department of Neurosurgery on time, early surgery (within 72 hours) was carried out. Early surgery was performed in all patients in a clinical state grade IV or V after Hunt and Hess, if the clinical state improved after insertion of an external ventricular drain. In case of missing clinical improval, surgery was delayed until the clinical state became better. Intraoperative Doppler sonography was used routinely to verify the patency of aneurysm-bearing vessels after clipping of the aneurysm. Transcranial Doppler sonography (TCD) was carried out daily in order to detect cerebral vasospasm on time. In case of a daily increase of blood flow velocity of more than 0.5 kHz, antiischemic treatment consisting of induced hypertension, moderate hypervolemia and hemodilution was

Table 1. Causes of mortality in a series of 390 microneurosurgically treated patients after the rupture of one or more intracranial aneurysms

Cause	No.	%
Initial bleeding	18	4,6
Operative complications	6	1,5
Vasospasm	4	1
Medical complications	4	1
Unknown	1	0,3
Postoperative mortality	33	8,4

According to Hütter et al. (1999)

initiated (Kreitschmann-Andermahr and Gilsbach, 1996). In patients with a critical amount of intraventricular blood, recombinant tissue plasminogen activator (rtPA) was applied intraventricularly via a ventricular catheter (Mayfrank et al., 1997a;b). Of the 390 patients operated upon, 33 (8.4%) died during a follow-up period of six months. Table 1 lists the different causes of death in the Aachen series.

In 6 (1.5%) patients, the fatal result could be attributed directly to surgery. Presumably due to the intravenous application of nimodipine (Barker and Ogilvy, 1996; Gilsbach et al., 1990), daily Doppler sonography (TCD) and modified triple "H"-therapy, only 1% of all fatalities are attributable directly to cerebral vasospasm. Of the remaining 32 patients with aneurysmal SAH in whom no indication for surgery was seen because of their poor clinical state, 25 (78%) died. This means that the total treatment mortality made up of the postoperative and non-operative fatalites amounted to 13.7% in the Aachen series (Hütter et al., 1999).

4. Special aspects of the pathology and therapy of SAH

4.1. The importance of the anatomical distribution of the hemorrhage

The wide distribution of CCT scanners has led to a faster and more reliable diagnosis of SAH. Furthermore, the possibility arose to determine the amount of blood and its anatomical distribution exactly. Therefore, a variety of methods has been proposed to measure the amount of blood after aneurysm rupture based on CCT. Sano, Kanno and Shinomiya (1982) measured the density of a given point in the subarachnoid space in Hounsfield units. Other research groups recorded the thickness of the blood layers in the basal cisterns (Forssell et al., 1995; Gurusinghe and Richardson, 1984; Fisher, Kistler and Davis, 1980). While some scoring systems only quantified the amount of blood in the basal cistern (Hasan and Tanghe, 1992; Hijdra et al., 1990; Gurusinghe and Richardson, 1984), the CCT grading system by Fisher, Kistler and Davis (1980) also takes the presence of intracerebral hematoma and/or intraventricular blood into consideration. On the other hand, the Fisher CCT grading confounds the amount of subarachnoid blood and the presence of intracerebral and/or intraventricular hematoma. However, a separate listing would be more desirable.

At present, the CCT scoring system of Fisher, Kistler and Davis (1980) is by far the most accepted method to quantify the severity of SAH on the basis of morphological criteria. In several studies, it proved to be a prognostically valid indicator for clinical course, mortality and morbidity in patients with SAH after aneurysm rupture (Hauerberg, Eskesen and Rosenorn, 1994; Gilsbach et al., 1988a; Adams, Kassell and Torner, 1985; Adams et al., 1983; Fisher, Kistler and Davis, 1980). On the other hand, the Fisher score as well as other grading systems that allow only a restricted number of categories is not suitable to evaluate the variability of the anatomical distribution and the amount of intracranial blood after SAH satisfactorily (Van Gijn et al., 1985a). A more differentiated method to assess the severity of SAH has been proposed by Hijdra et al. (1990), according to which the amount of blood is rated separately in 10 basal cisterns and fissures. Despite all weaknesses, a number of clinical studies underline the prognostic importance of the severity of the bleeding as assessed according to the initial CCT (Mayfrank, 1997; Shapiro, Campbell and Scully, 1994; Browers et al., 1993; Hütter and Gilsbach, 1993; Adams, Kassell and Torner, 1985; Gurusinghe and Richardson, 1984).

Detailed neuroanatomic topographic analysis of the neighboring anatomical structures of the basal cisterns reveals numerous regions that can also be regarded as particularly important for a great number of cognitive functions according to general neuropsychological knowledge (Hütter, 1997a; Hütter et al., 1997a;b; Hütter and Gilsbach, 1996a; Mesulam, 1985; Damasio et al., 1985b). Table 1 lists the respective basal cisterns and the neighboring anatomical structures of potential neuropsychological relevance.

It is a promising starting point for future research on the neuropsychological sequelae of SAH to differentiate the respective bleeding distribution according to the affected basal cisterns and the concerned neighboring anatomical structures in relationship to the pattern of cognitive deficits (Hütter et al., 1998; Hütter, Kreitschmann-Andermahr and Gilsbach, 1998). Even if direct empirical evidence for this hypothesis is still missing, it seems plausible when scrutinizing the list of the neighboring structures of the basal cisterns, that memory and attention deficits belong to the most frequent neuropsychological sequelae after SAH, since especially parts of the limbic system are situated in close vicinity to the basal cisterns (Hütter et al., 1997a;b; Mesulam, 1985).

Table 1. The basal cisterns and neighboring neuroanatomical structures of supposed neuropsychological relevance

Basal cistern	Related neuroanatomical structure(s)
C. carotis	Parts of the orbital frontal lobe Parts of the medial temporal lobe Uncus
C. laminae terminalis	Rostrum corpus callosi Gyrus rectus Commissura anterior
C. olfactorii	Parts of the orbital frontal lobe Gyrus rectus
C. fossa sylvii	Parts of the orbital frontal lobe Parts of the baso-medial temporal lobe Limen insulae
C. cruralis (interpeduncularis)	Parahippocampal gyrus
C. ambiens	Lateral sections of the tegmentum Cerebral peduncles Parts of the medial temporal lobe Uncus Velum interpositum Pulvinar thalami
C. vena magna Galeni	Dorsal sections of the tegmentum Splenium corporis callosi

Table 1 (*continued*)

C. velum interpositum	Splenium corporis callosi Fornix Pulvinar thalamiz
C. corpus callosi	Rostrum corpus callosi Cingulate gyrus Corpus callosum
C. interpeduncularis	Tegmentum Substantia perforata rostralis Mamillary bodies Parts of the medial temporal lobe
C. praepontina	Pons
C. medullaris anterior	Pons Medulla oblongata
C. cerebellopontina	Pons
C. cerebellomedullaris lateralis	Medulla oblongata
C. magna	Medulla oblongata

4.2. Intraventricular hemorrhage

Intraventricular hemorrhage (IVH) is present in up to 56% of all cases after aneurysm rupture (LeRoux et al., 1996a). It is important for the analysis of the neuropsychological sequelae of IVH in connection to SAH to consider the anatomical ways by means of which the blood can reach the ventricles: The first possibility involves the breakthrough of aneurysmal blood through the cerebral parenchyma into the ventricles. This happens most often, although not inevitably, during the rupture of an ACoA aneurysm when intracerebral hemorrhage occurs into the medial frontal lobe, oftentimes contralaterally, depending on the site of rupture. Since the cerebral parenchyma is very thin between an ACoA aneurysm and the frontal horn of the lateral ventricle, blood may enter the frontal horn of the lateral ventricle and the septum pellucidum. A second possibility for the blood to enter the ventricles after aneurysmal SAH involves a retrograde flow of blood from the basal cisterns into the fourth ventricle. A third mechanism is the direct aneurysmal hemorrhage into the ventricle, most often the case in PICA aneurysms or the much rarer intraventricular aneurysms. Figure 1, gratefully acknowledged to Prof. Seeger (Freiburg), who illustrated this relationship, gives a detailed overview of the anatomical site and the frontobasal cortical and subcortical structures involved in the route of entry of blood in the case of intraventricular hemorrhage (IVH) out of a ruptured ACoA aneurysm in this example. Aneurysms of other location may, however, cause IVH as well.

In the scientific literature, IVH has been identified as an important predictor of a bad neurological as well as neuropsychological outcome after SAH (Hütter, Kreitschmann-Andermahr and Gilsbach, 1998; Mayfrank, 1997; Kassell et al., 1990b; Adams, Kassell and Torner, 1985). According to the results of Hütter et al. (1999) and Mayfrank (1997), IVH was present on the initial CCT in 134 patients of 251 evaluated cases (53.4%) after SAH due to aneurysm rupture in the Aachen series. The severity of IVH was rated according to the system of Le Roux et al. (1992). Although the poor

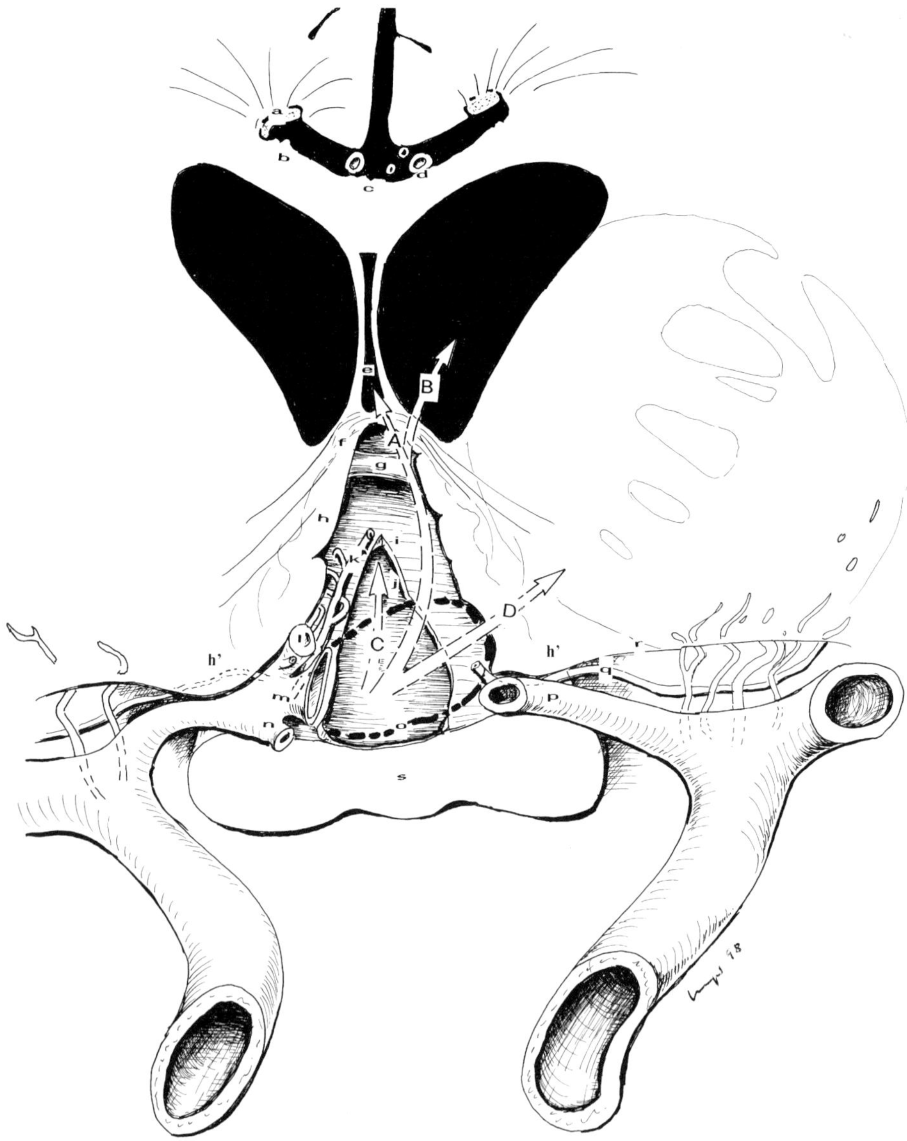

prognosis of patients with IVH may in part have been due to the association with a severe SAH, it was found that the presence of IVH was an independent predictor of mortality and morbidity in connection with SAH (Hütter et al., 1999; Mayfrank et al., 1997a;b; Mayfrank, 1997).

The mechanisms by which IVH may cause additional brain damage can be explained on the one hand by causing an acute hydrocephalus by obstructing the outflow pathways of cerebrospinal fluid (Van Gijn et al., 1985a; Mohr et al., 1983; Menon, Weir and Overton, 1981; Vassilouthis and Richardson, 1979). On the other hand, a compression of periventricular brain structures due to space-occupying intraventricular blood clots – especially in the fourth ventricle and the aqueduct – which may impede microcirculation can be presumed (Shapiro, Campbell and Scully, 1994). Both mechanisms can be counteracted by the intraventricular application of rtPA which accelerates clot clearance (Mayfrank, 1997; Mayfrank et al., 1997a;b; 1993). It can be hypothesized that fibrinolytic therapy can ameliorate the neurological, neuropsychological and psychosocial prognosis after IVH due to SAH (Hütter et al., 1999; Hütter, Kreitschmann-Andermahr and Gilsbach, 1998; Mayfrank, 1997; Mayfrank et al., 1997a;b; 1993; Rohde, Schaller and Hassler, 1995; Findlay, Grace and Weir, 1993).

4.3. Intracerebral hemorrhage

Intracerebral hemorrhage (ICH) is seen in up to 43% of patients after aneurysm rupture (Tokuda et al., 1995). Although aneurysms of any location may cause ICH, it is associated particularly with aneurysms of the MCA. Patients with ICH are in a significantly worse clinical state (Hunt and Hess) on arrival at a neurosurgical department as compared to those patients in whom the initial CCT did not demonstrate ICH (Tokuda et al., 1995; Adams et al., 1983). Damage to the cerebral parenchyma on the site of the hematoma, elevated intracranial pressure and secondary lesions of

Fig. 1. Anatomical situs according to Seeger demonstrating the four different main routes of the bleeding through the parenchyma in the case of an intraventricular hemorrhage (IVH). *a* Limbic cortex, cingular section of the stria lateralis; *b* as *a*, callosal section of the stria lateralis; *c* like *a* and *b*, stria medialis of the corpus callosum; *d* pericallosal a.; *e* cavum septi pellucidi; *f* fibers of the rostrum corporis callosi; *g* anterior commissure; *h* area subcallosa (mesocortical); *h′* gyrus rectus; *i* lamina terminalis (fenestrated); *j* 3rd ventricle (opened); *k* "anterior hypothalamic artery" (a. corporis callosi mediana, from n); *l* anterior cerebral a., distal part (so-called "A2"); *m* neck of the aneurysm; *n* anterior communicating a. (ACoA); *o* aneurysm (projection); *p* like l, proximal segment (so-called "A1"); *q* recurrent a. of Heubner; *r* anterior perforated substance; *s* chiasm. Arrows A to D: The four main routes of the bleeding through the parenchyma in the case of an IVH: *A* to the cavum septi pellucidi, *B* to the lateral ventricle, *C* to the 3rd ventricle and into the interhemispheric fissure (most frequent route) *D* into the parenchyma, here into the contralateral basal ganglia and into the posterior part of the gyrus rectus (frequent type)

the brainstem due to herniation of the uncus as well as the direct consequence of damage to the uncus represent the most important mechanisms by which ICH worsens the prognosis after SAH (Heiskanen et al., 1988). The estimation of the amount of subarachnoid, intraventricular and intracerebral blood after aneurysm rupture contains important prognostic information and is probably of considerable significance for the prognosis of mortality as well as the functional outcome.

5. Cerebral vasospasm after SAH

The introduction and worldwide application of the concept of early surgery after the rupture of an intracranial aneurysm as well as an improved intensive care management in the last two decades have contributed to a significant reduction of morbidity and mortality due to vasospasm. Fisher, Roberson and Ojemann (1977) found that 50% of 50 patients, who had survived SAH caused by aneurysm rupture, developed delayed neurological deficits as a consequence of vasospasm. In the Cooperative Study of Kassell et al. (1990a;b), 7.2% mortality and 6.3% permanent impairments were attributed to vasospasm. In the manifold literature on this topic, data on the incidence of vasospasm and the frequency of associated delayed ischemic deficits vary considerably. Various definitions of vasospasm and differences between the methods used to measure vasospasm are also responsible for the discrepancies.

However, according to the opinion of Hütter et al. (1999), Kreitschmann-Andermahr and Gilsbach (1996), as well as Hütter and Gilsbach (1993), the importance of symptomatic vasospasm as the cause for a bad neurological or neuropsychological outcome is probably overestimated. Many postoperative complications, appearing as delayed neurological deterioration are often falsely attributed to vasospasm (Compton, Redmond and Symon, 1987). Rather, other causes such as operative injuries and their indirect consequences, infections, electrolyte or metabolic disturbances, the SAH-associated syndromes of salt and water wasting, dysbalance of the secretion of antidiuretic hormone (SIADH), disturbances of CSF circulation up to hydrocephalus as well as brain edema must be taken into account.

The incidence of significantly increased blood flow velocities as a sign of vasospasm of more than 120 cm/s as measured by TCD amounts to 70–75% in patients after aneurysm rupture (Harders and Gilsbach, 1987). In reality, only some of these patients develop symptomatic vasospasm. Nevertheless, TCD is the only screening method that allows to identify patients at risk to develop severe vasospasm in the asymptomatic stage and, therefore, constitutes the essential prerequisite for the initiation of early preventive hemodynamic therapy. An indirect advantage of early aneurysm surgery is that it provides the basic requirements for an adequate pharmacological management of vasospasm and also has a preventive effect by the diminution of the amount of subarachnoid blood. The apprehension that the surgical trauma of early surgery would negate these advantages can meanwhile be regarded as baseless, also from a neuropsychological point of view (Hütter et al., 1999; Hütter, Kreitschmann-Andermahr and Gilsbach,

1998; Hütter and Gilsbach, 1996a; Hütter, Gilsbach and Kreitschmann-Andermahr, 1995; Kreitschmann-Andermahr, Hütter and Gilsbach, 1995; Hütter, Gilsbach and Kreitschmann, 1994; Gilsbach and Harders, 1989).

The treatment regimen for the prevention and treatment of secondary ischemic deficits due to vasospasm, applied in the Department of Neurosurgery, University Hospital of the University of Technology (RWTH) Aachen, is essentially founded on pharmacologically induced hypertension as the most important and most effective component of triple "H"-therapy. Hypervolemia, hemodilution and hypertension (triple "H"-therapy) are used to ameliorate cerebral perfusion by means of the elevation of perfusion pressure (Kreitschmann-Andermahr and Gilsbach, 1996; Gilsbach and Harders, 1989). Triple "H"-therapy must be initiated at the latest upon the beginning of symptomatic ischemic deficits. However, it is much more effective when a preventive regimen is begun according to TCD criteria when patients are still in the asymptomatic stage (Kreitschmann-Andermahr and Gilsbach, 1996; Gilsbach et al., 1990; Gilsbach and Harders, 1989; Gilsbach, 1988; Harders and Gilsbach, 1987). Moreover, a consequent pharmacological therapy with the calcium antagonist nimodipine is performed.

In a retrospective pilot study, Kreitschmann-Andermahr, Hütter and Gilsbach (1996; 1995) investigated the effectiveness of aggressive catecholamine-induced hypertension in combination with hypervolemia for the treatment of severe prolonged vasospasm after SAH, defined as elevated mean blood flow velocities (TCD) of more than 160 cm/s on five consecutive days after SAH. A total of 15 patients had been treated by means of catecholamine-induced hypertension. 12 further patients, who had received a comparable surgical and medical treatment without catecholamine therapy served as the control group. Both groups did not differ in terms of age, sex, preoperative state according to Hunt and Hess, severity of the bleeding (Fisher CCT Score) and the average duration of vasospasm ($p > 0.05$, respectively). In analogy to the treatment concept, systolic blood pressure during the phase of vasospasm was significantly higher in the catecholamine group ($p < 0.000$). The neurological outcome was rated upon discharge from the department according to the Glasgow Outcome Scale (GOS) by an investigator, who had, at that time point, no information on the pharmacological regimen applied on the intensive care ward. Moreover, the HRQOL of the surviving patients was rated after an average of 28 months using two questionnaires (Aachen Quality of Life Inventory, ALQI), one for self-assessment and a parallel version for assessment by the life-companion of the patient (Hütter and Gilsbach, 1996b;1995b).

Two patients in the catecholamine group died of vasospastic infarction. No further patient in this group developed structural lesions visible on CCT as a consequence of vasospasm. In the control group, one patient died of vasospastic infarction and two further patients developed infarcts seen on CCT and attributed to vasospasm. At discharge, 11 (73%) patients in the catecholamine group were in a good neurological state (GOS = I), the remaining two patients were rated as GOS = II. In the non-catecholamine

Table 1. Quality of life of patients after severe prolonged vasospasm after SAH

ALQI Summary scores of impairment	Catecholamine group		Control group		t-test
	Mean	SD	Mean	SD	p
ALQI Physical Score (self-rating)	3,6	4,6	6,5	5,8	0,09 ns
ALQI Psycho-social Score (self-rating)	6,5	5,8	11,5	9,7	0,09 ns
ALQI Total score (self-rating)	15,5	12,3	25,5	15,1	0,07 ns
ALQI Total score (proxy-rating)	12,7	9,4	30,7	18,7	0,01*

ALQI = Aachen Life Quality Inventory; SD = standard deviation; ns = not significant; *$p < 0,05$. Acccording to Kreitschmann-Andermahr, Hütter and Gilsbach (1996; 1995)

group, five (42%) patients presented with a good neurological result (GOS = I), in three (25%) patients the neurological result had been estimated as GOS = II and a further three (25%) patients had sustained a severe neurological deficit (GOS = III). The difference in the degree of neurological impairment with a tendency toward a better result in the catecholamine group was statistically only nearly significant ($p = 0.06$). In terms of the later quality of life, the catecholamine-treated patients presented with significantly less impairments in the ALQI subscales mobility ($p = 0.02$) and freetime activities ($p = 0.04$). On the other hand, according to the results of the patients' self-assessment, no statistically significant differences in the total number of impairments and the sum scores of the psychosocial and physical aspects of quality of life between both groups emerged. There was a trend, however, toward a lesser degree of impairment in the catecholamine group (Table 1). From the perspective of the patients' life-companions, the patients in the treatment group were significantly less impaired that those who had not been treated by catecholamine-induced hypertension (Table 1).

This retrospective pilot study compared two concepts for the treatment of severe prolonged vasospasm after SAH (Kreitschmann-Andermahr, Hütter and Gilsbach, 1995; 1996). Although trends in favor of the catecholamine group could be demonstrated, the differences in the neurological state (GOS) at discharge from the department and in terms of self-rated quality of life after an average of 28 months did not reach statistical significance. Since the sample size of this pilot study is relatively small, the power of the therapeutic effect is not sufficient to substantiate the observed differences on a statistical basis. Further limitations result of the small group sizes, that diminish the conclusions that can be drawn from the results. Mortality and the number of observed vasospastic infarcts in both groups are absolutely to small for statistical comparison. Therefore, the pilot study of Kreitschmann-Andermahr, Hütter and Gilsbach (1995; 1996) can be regarded at most as an indicator for the potential effectiveness of catecholamine treatment. It is

Table 1. Neurological result according to the GOS at discharge from the neurosurgical unit of n = 76 patients who were on admission in grade IV or V (Hunt and Hess grading)

Neurological result at discharge	Grade IV (n = 44)		Grade V (n = 32)	
	n	%	n	%
Good (GOS = I)	10	23	4	13
Fair (GOS = II)	10	23	8	25
Bad (GOS = III–IV)	17	39	8	25
Dead (GOS = V)	7	16	12	38

GOS = Glasgow Outcome Scale (Jennett and Bond, 1967)

Table 2. Neurological result according to the GOS 8 months after discharge from the hospital of n = 76 patients who were on admission in grade IV or V (Hunt and Hess grading)

Neurological result 8 months after discharge	Grade IV (n = 44)		Grade V (n = 32)	
	n	%	n	%
Good (GOS = I)	16	36	8	25
Fair (GOS = II)	13	30	4	13
Bad (GOS = III–IV)	6	14	8	25
Dead (GOS = V)	9	20	12	38

GOS = Glasgow Outcome Scale (Jennett and Bond, 1967)

treatment on average after 23 days and the late result at follow-up at a mean of 8 months after the intervention. The results of this study (according to the GOS) are represented in Tables 1 and 2.

The overall neurological late result after early surgery in patients in a neurological state grade IV or V after Hunt and Hess was favorable in 41 (54%) patients (GOS = I or II) and unfavorable in 35 (46%) patients (GOS III to V). Immediate postoperative deterioration could be attributed to surgical problems such as massive hemorrhage (1%) due to premature aneurysm rupture, prolonged temporary clipping (3%), occlusion of a large perforating vessel (4%) and to damage of small perforators or their injury caused by local compression due to spatula pressure (5%). The incision of the lamina terminalis is important to facilitate the circulation of CSF, especially in patients in a poor clinical state who are at a larger risk to develop hydrocephalus at a later point of time. Set apart from the overall mortality in this patient group, the frequency of postoperatively permanently and severely impaired patients must be considered from a neuropsychological point of view. Of all patients in Hunt and Hess grades IV or V, 18% of the Aachen patients remained in a poor neurological state according to the GOS (GOS = IV) with severe impairments associated with the entire complexity of medical, psychological, ethical and financial problems of long-time nursing and life-long intense care. The result that 46% of all patients in this series exhibited an unfavorable clinical result, i.e. died or remained severely impaired, cannot be generally attributed to surgical damage, but to the adverse course of the underlying illness. However, the question of the later quality of life of the surviving patients, especially those in an initial Hunt and Hess grade IV or V, remains. Not only the later quality of life of those patients who have survived the operative procedure and later complications remains to be elucidated. Moreover, additional criteria must be formulated that might be important indicators for maximal therapy in this patient group.

7. Neuropsychological sequelae of SAH

7.1. Early studies on the neuropsychological sequelae of SAH

7.1.1. Single case studies and unsystematic case reports

Due to the considerable changes that have evolved in aneurysm surgery and treatment of SAH since the seventies, also the neuropsychological studies completed before that time are not comparable to later investigations. It is sensible, therefore, to present and to discuss the former apart from the more recent studies, conducted since the late nineteen seventies. Based on the substantial differences between the individual clinical departments, it can neither be taken for granted, however, that in all studies published since the nineteen eighties, microneurosurgical methods have been used consistently, nor that the respective units are comparable in terms of surgical, pharmacological and intensive care management of SAH.

Early reports on the neuropsychological sequelae of SAH consist for the most part of single case studies or unsystematic collections of case reports. Those patients after the rupture of an ACoA aneurysm prevail, whereas investigations on the neuropsychological sequelae of the rupture of aneurysms of other locations are to be found much more infrequently. The largest disadvantage of case reports consists in the account of selected individual cases which must not be representative for a given sample or diagnostic group. This is in so far dangerous as that untypical exceptions, selected according to a certain criterion, are exposed. In extreme cases, the selected trait may only be present coincidentally in a single patient of a certain diagnostic group. This danger is present even more so if the clinical and neuroradiological documentation of the patient is incomplete or even erroneous. Therefore, generalized conclusions, drawn from the findings of case studies and applied to a population of patients suffering from a certain illness are not warranted and, moreover, are associated with the risk of misleading interpretations. A plastic example herefore is given by the early studies on Korsakoff's syndrome in patients with a ruptured ACoA aneurysm. In larger series, the incidence of Korsakoff psychosis after the rupture of an ACoA aneurysm ranges around 3% since the early days of aneurysm surgery (David, Pertuiset and Guyot, 1968; Walton, 1953; Tarachow, 1939). Moreover, Korsakoff psychosis is by no means a typical symptom of a ruptured ACoA aneurysm, as suggested by the numerous case reports, but also occurs after the rupture of aneurysms of other locations (Norlen, 1975). Individual reports even show a tendency toward a larger frequency of

Korsakoff psychosis after ruptured aneurysms of other locations than the ACoA (Nyström, 1973).

A further disadvantage of many older papers lies in the fact that no systematic neuropsychological or neuropsychiatric investigation had been performed and only an unsystematic description of the symptoms was given. Also, the terminology in many publications is old-fashioned and does not comply to the modern use of the language. This may lead to misunderstandings and false interpretations. Moreover, as a rule, details on morphological brain damage and on the course of the illness that are verified by modern diagnostic methods are missing. From a present point of view, in the surgically treated patients most traumatic techniques had been used, whose effects are neither documented from the morphological side nor can they be separated from the sequelae of the SAH itself. This problem also exists for the secondary brain damage as a consequence of the hemorrhage.

The first description in the broadest sense of the neuropsychological sequelae of SAH stems from Hamilton Roe, who documented in 1852 the case of a 21 year-old woman who had been treated in Westminster Hospital on January 7th, 1851 because of blindness on the right eye and a memory loss for events in the near past (Roe, 1852). After her death on March 11th, 1851, autopsy revealed a thrombosed aneurysm of the size of a walnut above the sella turcica (Roe, 1852). Already in 1866, Hermann Lebert advanced the opinion that the respective localization of an intracranial aneurysm was associated with specific neurological and mental deficits (Lebert, 1866). Therefore, Lebert speculated that the localization of the aneurysm could be surmised from the clinical symptomatology (Lebert, 1866). Mental abnormalities with or without visual disturbances point, according to Lebert (1866) to an aneurysm of a segment of the anterior circulation. It is noteworthy, that this is the first time that the hypothesis of specific mental symptoms dependent on the location of the respective aneurysm is forwarded in the scientific literature.

Also as a result of the first advances of diagnostics and therapy of SAH, the number of publications on the mental sequelae of SAH increased markedly during the twenties of the twentieth century. Oftentimes, the psychological abnormalities after SAH were described as a Korsakoff psychosis (Walton, 1953; Tarachow, 1939; Cubbitt, 1930; Hall, 1929; Hermann, 1925; Goldflam, 1923; Flateau, 1921). The symptoms were described as fluctuating. While apathy was regarded to dominate during the acute stage according to the authors, euphoria, instable mood, general disorientation, global anterograde amnesia and diverse degrees of retrograde amnesias followed subsequently (Walton, 1953; Tarachow, 1939; Cubbitt, 1930; Hall, 1929; Hermann, 1925; Goldflam, 1923; Flateau, 1921). Disorientation and confabulation were described as typically subsiding within days or weeks, whereas emotional changes and memory impairments persisted for a longer period of time. It was reported that some patients attained their old normal self again, some slowly, others abruptly (Walton, 1953; Tarachow, 1939; Cubbitt, 1930; Hall, 1929; Hermann, 1925; Goldflam,

1923; Flateau, 1921). However, in none of the cited studies, the cause of SAH or the extent and kind of organic brain damage is specified. In some cases, autopsies were able to demonstrate a ruptured aneurysm as the cause of the bleeding. Since none of the patients described in these publications had been operated upon, the observed psychological abnormalities must be regarded as sequelae of the hemorrhage itself and associated secondary complications.

For one of the first cases of successful aneurysm surgery, an even for those times relatively detailed description of the psychopathological symptoms in the afflicted patient exists, including the pre- and postoperative course (Nattras, 1928). A 52 year-old woman had sustained a sudden severe headache in combination with vomiting six weeks prior to admission to the Royal Victoria Infirmary in Newcastle Upon-Tyne, which had been interpreted as the clinical signs of SAH. Already two to three years earlier, the patient had become symptomatic with a psychoorganic syndrome characterized by loquaciousness, euphoria and monotonous sing-song. Nattras (1928) interpreted these symptoms as the expression of frontal brain damage. The suspected ICA aneurysm in the left cavernous sinus was excluded from circulation surgically by ligature of the ICA at the neck of the aneurysm. No new symptoms emerged immediately postoperatively and the psychopathological disturbances remitted completely within one year (Nattrass, 1928). The brain organic substrate for this psychoorganic syndrome and its remittance remain unfortunately unresolved and the causes for postoperative improvement of the psychopathological abnormalities cannot be reconstructed on the basis of this case report. It is likely, however, that a further prior SAH was the cause for the primary disturbances of the patient.

Interestingly, in connection with the first early surgery in the history of aneurysm surgery, conducted by Dott on April 22nd 1931, it is reported that the patient was aphasic already preoperatively (Dott, 1933). Surgery took place two days after a 53 year-old man had sustained his third SAH due to the rupture of a left-sided aneurysm of the MCA. The aneurysm was "wrapped", as it was enveloped in muscle tissue as completely as possible. No new deficits emerged postoperatively and the aphasia may have recovered completely as a considerable recuperation of the patient within the following two years has been reported. This recovery was so far-reaching that the patient did not exhibit "any blatant signs of brain damage" two years later (Dott, 1933). Unfortunately, neither systematic neuropsychological methods had been applied, nor is the description of the symptomatology and the clinical course unequivocal. Further interesting case reports on the neuropsychological sequelae of the surgical methods for the exclusion of aneurysms common at the time also stem from Dott (1933). Dott operated on four patients with ruptured aneurysms of the left ICA. Preoperatively all patients had been aphasic, which leads to the assumption that the rupture of a left-sided ICA aneurysm is associated with a higher risk for an aphasic language disturbance. The techniques used by Dott (1933) for the exclusion of the aneurysm from circulation consisted in the "wrapping" with muscle tissue in one case and in the ligature of the ICA proximal to the site of rupture in the other cases. In two of the patients operated upon, the aphasia remitted, whereas it persisted in the other two (Dott, 1933).

Taren (1965) reported on a patient who exhibited a confused and disorientated behavior three years after the ligature of an ACoA aneurysm. A detailed description of the neuropsychological symptomatology and objective test psychological findings are, however, missing. During the course of surgery it had become necessary to detach the aneurysm from the basal frontal lobe structures such as the parolfactory region (Taren, 1965). Since the author suspected this aspect of the intervention to be responsible for the persisting abnormalities in his patient, he set in his opinion roughly comparable lesions in the brains of seven macaques. The monkeys were sacrificed after 17 days for histological analysis. Unanimously, the preparations showed a degeneration of the septum, the tuberculo-septo-hippocampal pathways, the cingulum, the fornix and the hippocampus (Taren, 1965). From this, the author concluded that in his patient with a ruptured ACoA aneurysm, damage to the septum had led to the persisting brain organic psychosyndrome.

The first reports on the neuropsychological sequelae of aneurysmal SAH, in which a systematic diagnostic assessment with standardized procedures had been applied, originate in the nineteen sixties. In those studies, the psychological sequelae of the rupture and surgical elimination exclusively of ACoA aneurysms were investigated (Norlen and Lindquist, 1964; Brion et al., 1968; Talland, Sweet and Ballantine, 1967). Norlen and Lindquist (1964) reported on 14 patients with a ruptured ACoA aneurysm who had been investigated psychiatrically and by means of psychometric tests. In 9 (64%) patients, a Korsakoff syndrome was diagnosed. In one patient the Korsakoff syndrome already emerged as a consequence of the bleeding, in the other patients immediately after surgery. In the course of several months, the symptomatology was reversible in six patients spontaneously, whereas it persisted permanently in three patients. Norlen and Lindquist (1964) speculated that structures of critical importance for memory functions must have been damaged. This could, on the one side, have been caused by interruption of the blood supply to these structures due to the ligature of vessels during surgery. The immediate damage of brain tissue by the hemorrhage itself, by spatula pressure during surgery or the preparation or dissection of the aneurysm, respectively, were suspected as further causes (Norlen and Lindquist, 1964).

Even to the present day, the case report of Talland, Sweet and Ballantine, (1967) belongs to the much cited "classical" publications in this area. The authors conducted repeated neuropsychological examinations over a time period of four years in two patients after the rupture of and surgery on an ACoA aneurysm. Both patients were substantially confused and disorientated before surgery. After the intervention, details of which are unfortunately missing, both patients were described as awake and cooperative. A formal neuropsychological testing revealed a normal memory span. On the other side, disorientation and confabulation remained. Beyond this, in both patients an anterograde amnesia was present. One of the two patients was able to return to work after a little more than half a year post surgery, although not in his old profession. The other patient remained unable to work, for the most part on the ground of a substantial lack of initiative. Both patients sustained permanent changes of personality, one became depressive while the other showed an inadequate good mood up to euphoria. Talland, Sweet and Ballantine (1967) attributed these abnormalities to bilateral damage to the mamillary bodies and the dorsomedial thalamus, perhaps due to bilateral ischemia. This interpretation is not founded, however, on manifest morphological brain damage verified by imaging diagnostics, but rather on the similarities to the Wernicke-Korsakoff-syndrome, which had been observed by the authors in both patients (Talland 1965; 1960). Based on intraoperative findings, it was postulated that both patients exhibited smaller lesions in posterior inferior medial frontal areas (Talland, Sweet and Ballantine, 1967). This terminology does not help to clarify, however, which anatomical structures exactly were involved.

Brion et al. (1968) report in detail on two cases of a Korsakoff syndrome, which they observed in their patients in a total of 3 (12.5%) of 24 patients operated upon an aneurysm of the anterior circulation. The first patient recovered relatively well from his SAH and was operated upon three weeks later on an ACoA aneurysm. During the intervention, parts of both gyri recti had to be resected. Clipping of the aneurysm was not possible so that in the end it had to be "wrapped" with muscle tissue. Although the immediate postoperative state of the patient was described as "subnormal", on the sixth postoperative day a severe brain organic syndrome occurred which became better gradually. However, four months later a Korsakoff syndrome associated with a disturbance of spatial orientation and inappropriate behavior was still present (Brion et al., 1968). An explanation for this sudden drastic decompensation of the patient is not provided by the authors. It may be speculated, however, that apart from the direct consequences of surgery such as the bilateral resection of the gyrus rectus and damage to the perforating arteries originating from the ACoA, delayed vasospasm or a disturbance of cerebrospinal fluid resorption accounts for the clinical state. The second case of a postoperative Korsakoff syndrome presented by Brion et al. (1968) emerged after clipping of an ACoA aneurysm, although both Aa. anteriores had been left intact according to angiographic criteria. A follow-up investigation three years after the intervention showed a remittance of the Korsakoff syndrome, however, a severely disturbed short-time memory and an anterograde amnesia for all events since surgery was still present, pointing to a considerable impairment also of long-term memory functions.

Luria (1976) gave account of a systematic neuropsychological investigation of two patients with a ruptured ACoA aneurysm. Both patients were examined almost daily neuropsychologically during a two-month postoperative course. A further patient was examined neuropsychologically one year after surgery on an ACoA aneurysm (Luria, 1976). Already preoperatively, all three patients had in common that they presented with considerable psychological alterations and especially a (modality-unspecific) amnestic syndrome, which also persisted postoperatively. The only new deficit that emerged postoperatively was a markedly increased distractibility and susceptibility for interference in both patients (Luria, 1976). Luria (1976) noted on the ground of his clinical experience that these patients, in contrary to amnestics with deep structural brain lesions, i.e. due to a tumor, did not exhibit a global alteration of consciousness or a decreased vigilance. Luria (1976) attempted to explain for himself gradual differences in the abnormalities in ACoA patients (amnestic syndrome with or without confabulations, emotional changes and decreased introspection and an exclusive amnestic syndrome without any other neuropsychological or neuropsychiatric alterations) by means of fine differences in the main region of the morphological brain damage (Luria, 1976). Yet, these hypotheses of Luria (1976) must be regarded as highly speculative, since in no patient imaging diagnostics exist which should have revealed morphological brain damage. Moreover, the complex clinical entity of SAH is not suitable for differentiated functional-anatomical deliberations.

A further case report is provided by Stuss et al. (1978), who gave account of five patients showing an unusual and persisting variant of confabulations. These were characterized particularly by spontaneous, lasting and especially unrealistic up to distinctly fantastic confabulations. Two of these patients had survived SAH due to the rupture of an ACoA aneurysm. The other patients, two of which were chronic alcoholics, had sustained severe head injury. The first SAH patient had been operated upon four weeks after the acute hemorrhage. Preoperatively, he presented neither with amnestic nor neurological deficits. Immediately postoperatively, a slight hemiparesis and an apathetic confused state occurred. CCT performed six weeks later showed a large right-sided fronto-medial infarction, whereas angiography demonstrated the occlusion of the right ACA. The stupor had abated at that time, but a pronounced Korsakoff syndrome with numerous confabulations which showed no tendency for remittance over four months, had taken its place. The other patient in the case study by Stuss et al. (1978) showed an uneventful postoperative course after the rupture and surgical exclusion of an ACoA aneurysm and could be discharged home in a good clinical state. Seven months later he developed progressive states of confusion, confabulations, sexual disinhibition and anosognosia, accompanied by intermitting incontinence. The other neurological findings were normal. These characteristics of the clinical course lead to the assumption of secondary acute hydrocephalus. Also after implantation of a ventriculo-peritoneal shunt, the state of the patient did not improve. Stuss et al. (1978) report, however, on the radiological finding of an extensive frontal porencephalic cyst. The confabulatory symptoms were explained by Stuss et al. (1978) using a two-component theory, according to which a severe memory impairment is overlapped by an even more pronounced disturbance of frontal lobe functions.

However, these early findings document unanimously that cognitive, motivational and emotional changes may persist after SAH, whereas in the area of cognitive impairments memory disturbances are in the forefront of these deficits. It is noticeable, that many descriptions concern a Korsakoff syndrome, emerging after SAH or aneurysm surgery. However, even under the medical management conditions of that time, this entity must have been the exception from the rule. Walton (1953) and Tarachow (1939), respectively, estimated the incidence of Korsakoff psychosis as a consequence of SAH at 2–3%. Furthermore, it is remarkable that in many patients already preoperatively neuropsychological and neuropsychiatric alterations existed, which points to the causal importance of the bleeding and events associated therewith. The description of postoperative improvements of the preoperative symptomatology leads to conclude that the surgical intervention was seemingly not always associated with additional damage to the patient. On the other hand, at present, the causes for such improvements cannot be clarified anymore and must, therefore, remain speculative.

7.1.2. Early group studies on the neuropsychological sequelae of SAH

Also the great majority of group studies in the time before 1980 concern the neuropsychological sequelae of the rupture and operative exclusion from circulation of an ACoA aneurysm. Apart from the oftentimes observed brain organic psychosyndromes such as Korsakoff-like amnesias in this patient group, the lack of interest for other aneurysm locations can probably be traced back to an up to now prevalent misconception. This consists in the assumption that the neuropsychological deficits after the rupture of an aneurysm are identical to those occurring after vascular occlusive disease of the aneurysm-bearing vessel or intracranial hemorrhage. The limitations discussed for single case studies like the lack of a formal neurological or neuropsychiatric clinical investigation, insufficient data on morphological brain damage and on the course of the illness or the application of old-fashioned surgical techniques, also hold true for the majority of group studies. In so far, these older studies are not comparable to recent ones.

One of the first group studies including a systematic neuropsychological investigation of the patients was performed by Lindquist and Norlen (1966). The study group consisted of 33 patients who had been operated upon after the rupture of an ACoA aneurysm. In 30 patients surgical treatment consisted of the ligature of the neck of the aneurysm or the application of the "trapping" procedure. In one patient, the neck of the aneurysm had been excluded together with the parent vessel (ACoA) by means of electrocoagulation, whereas in the other two cases, the aneurysm was wrapped using synthetic material. Seventeen (50%) patients developed a Korsakoff syndrome in the acute postoperative stage, accompanied by emotional indifference. In five (15%) patients, the Korsakoff syndrome persisted permanently (Lindquist and Norlen, 1966). David, Pertuiset and Guyot (1968) found a postoperative Korsakoff syndrome in only 3 (3%) of 99 patients with an ACoA aneurysm. However, David, Pertuiset and Guyot (1968) did not use a standardized neuropsychological and/or neuropsychiatric assessment in their study.

Storey (1970; 1967) published a psychiatric follow-up investigation of 261 patients between six months and six years after the rupture of an ACoA, MCA or PCoA aneurysm. The patients had been assigned according to a randomized design either to a conservative or operative treatment group. Neurosurgical techniques included either the ligature of the carotid artery, "direct" exclusion of the aneurysm (most likely wrapping or ligature of the neck of the aneurysm) and the proximal exclusion of the aneurysm-bearing vessel, which was applied exclusively in ACoA aneurysms. In 30 patients, an aneurysm could not be demonstrated angiographically. Only 45% of the patients were evaluated as psychiatrically normal, whereas in 21% a moderate to severe psychiatric abnormality was found. Lesser symptoms such as a lowered incentive, increased irritability and anxiety were diagnosed in 55% of the patients. Personality disorders were highly significantly ($p < 0.0001$) associated with the severity of neurological impairments. An association with the location of the aneurysm was, however, not found. Severe abnormalities like depression, substantially increased emotional lability and anxiety were significantly more pronounced in MCA aneurysm patients with a trend in the direction of more severe impairments in right-sided as compared to left-sided MCA aneurysms. Psychiatric morbidity in the MCA group was significantly higher in the operated patients than in the conservatively treated, which indicates the considerable technical problems of surgery of MCA aneurysms at that time. Socially inadequate behavior, loquaciousness and agitation were, in comparison to other patients, significantly more pronounced after the rupture of an ACoA aneurysm.

Patients after the rupture of a PCoA aneurysm exhibited significantly less personality disorders that all other patients (Storey, 1970; 1967). Although patients without a proven aneurysm exhibited a significantly lower neurological morbidity, the incidence of psychiatric disturbances was equal in both groups. On the other hand, the results of Storey (1970; 1967) are strongly limited because considerable differences between the groups existed which, strictly spoken, forbade comparison. Apart from the lack of consideration of the severity of the bleeding, the initial clinical state and course (i.e. vasospasm), completely different and incomparable surgical techniques had been applied, especially in the patient groups with aneurysms of different locations (Storey, 1970; 1967). In so far, possible effects of aneurysm location are confounded with the effects of different surgical techniques in the study of Storey (1970; 1967).

In a follow-up study by Logue et al. (1968) 79 patients were investigated meticulously neurologically, neuropsychologically and by means of a psychiatric interview between 7 and 101 months after the rupture and surgical treatment of an ACoA aneurysm. In all operations, the ACA had been clipped proximally to the aneurysm. It is, however, likely, that already the occlusion of only one major branch of the ACA had led to an impaired perfusion of extensive frontal areas and, therefore, to cognitive deficits. Of the 79 investigated patients (66 surgically and 13 conservatively treated), 23 (29%) exhibited severe memory impairments. It was observed that short-term memory was overall more impaired than general intelligence. The group means in the Wechsler Intelligence Test corresponded to the expected value that represents the average performance level of the general public. Also, no differences between side of surgery or between operated and conservatively treated patients were found. At follow-up, in 32 (40.5%) patients, abnormalities were found at psychometrical testing that pointed to an aphasic language disturbance. A further result that is interesting in the light of modern attention theories consists in the fact that 24 (30%) of all patients reported to feel overstrained when more than two persons were engaged in conversation, which is an indicator for a substantially impaired attention capacity. Eighteen (22.7%) patients reported an increased susceptibility for interference, whereas loquaciousness was observed in 21 (26.5%) patients. A lowered initiative as a sequelae of the SAH was complained of by 48 (607%) patients. A further 30 (37.9%) patients noticed an impairment of emotional control mechanisms. Moreover, in a third of the patients, personality changes in the direction of increased carefreeness and euphoric mood were registered (Logue et al., 1968).

Lindquist conducted an extensive study in which 310 surgically treated patients after SAH were investigated on the frequency of Korsakoff syndrome and emotional-motivational changes after the rupture of an ACoA, MCA and ICA aneurysm (Lindquist, 1975; Norlen, 1975). In the early postoperative stage, in 37% of the ACoA patients, but only in 1% of the ACA and 4% of the MCA patients, a Korsakoff syndrome was diagnosed. Brain organic personality changes without Korsakoff syndrome were slightly higher in the ACoA group (11%), but also occurred in 9% of the MCA and 6% of the ICA patients (Norlen, 1975). The results of a study of Sengupta, Chinu and Brierley (1975) are in many ways different from the majority of earlier investigations. Between 4 and 33 months after surgical exclusion of an ACoA aneurysm, 26 patients were followed up by means of the Wechsler Intelligence Test, the Wechsler Memory Scale as well as a questionnaire on the basis of which the life companions of the patients had to rate the psychological adjustment of the patients. All operations had been performed without the use of a microscope and under controlled hypotension. In the vast majority of the interventions, it was attempted to clip the aneurysm at the neck, preserving the perforating vessels. In no patient, a persisting Korsakoff syndrome occurred. The mean test scores of the ACoA patients in the Wechsler Intelligence Test as well as the Wechsler Memory Scale corresponded exactly to the mean scores according to the test norms, although the relatives of 11 patients had observed a worsening of memory functions in these patients.

On the other side, the life companions reported of personality changes in the patients consisting of a loss of interests and initiative and of a lowered incentive. Unfortunately, Sengupta, Chinu and Brierley (1975) did not give quantitative specifications on these observations. However, patients with personality changes showed lower IQ-mean values than those who had been rated by their life companions as unchanged. Patients operated upon late were more impaired than those operated upon early. Numerous and significant correlations in a size of $r = 0.39$ to $r = 0.65$ between personality changes as loss of interests, lack of initiative and will power as well as decreased drive on the one hand and severity of the bleeding, preoperative clinical state and the severity of preoperative vasospasm were found (Sengupta, Chinu and Brierley, 1975). These results demonstrate that the psychological changes in the wake of aneurysmal SAH are predominantly the expression of the severity of the bleeding and associated secondary complications.

In further neurosurgical studies, the incidence of amnestic syndromes in patients after the rupture and surgical therapy of an intracranial aneurysm was investigated without formal neuropsychological testing or neuropsychiatric diagnostics. The concurrent observations consisted in the result that amnestic syndromes were more frequent in ACoA patients than in patients with ruptured aneurysms of other locations (Okawa et al., 1980; Takaku et al., 1979; David et al., 1968; Norlen and Olivecrona, 1953). Takaku et al. (1979) report that in their patients at the time of discharge from hospital, disorientation and amnesia were four times as frequent (14%) after the rupture of an ACoA aneurysm than in patients with a ruptured ACA, ICA or MCA aneurysm, with an average of 3.7% of such psychological changes at discharge. In contrast to the above cited authors, Nyström (1973) found a higher incidence of Korsakoff syndrome in patients with a left-sided ICA aneurysm than in patients after the rupture and operation of an ACoA aneurysm. In the cases investigated neuropsychologically, in 2 of 9 patients with a left-sided MCA aneurysm but only in 3 of 38 ACoA patients, a Korsakoff syndrome was found (Nyström, 1973). None of the patients with a ruptured right-sided MCA, or left- or right-sided ACA aneurysm showed a Korsakoff syndrome postoperatively. On the basis of the results of autopsies of some fatal MCA cases, Nyström (1973) conjectured that bilateral temporal damage due to hematoma and edema had led to the amnesia in patients with a ruptured left-sided MCA aneurysm (Nyström, 1973). Apart from the limited predictability of such casuistics, the autopsies described by Nyström (1973) underline that the localization of the factual macroscopic morphological brain damage and the side as well as the location of an intracranial aneurysm must not necessarily exhibit a clear association.

Almost all studies in the scientific literature concern themselves with the cognitive and emotional or psychiatric sequelae of SAH as well as the surgical repair of ruptured aneurysms. Penrose and Storey (1970) investigated just the opposite question, if and in how far emotional disturbances were not the consequence, but the cause of SAH. In a series of 261 patients after SAH due to aneurysm rupture and 30 patients after SAH without an angiographically proven source of the bleeding, Penrose and Storey (1970)

neuropsychology. Thus, in the study of Anderson, Tranel and Damasio (1988) all 10 patients after unilateral left-hemispheric cerebrovascular occlusive disease were aphasic, whereas only 4 out of 10 patients with brain tumors of comparable localization exhibited a, moreover only mild, aphasia. Meanwhile, it can be regarded as fact that considerable differences in the neuropsychological sequelae between cerebrovascular occlusive disease and brain tumors exist (Anderson, Tranel and Damasio, 1988; Mesulam, 1986; Parsons and Prigatano, 1978). The significance of the etiology of brain damage is so far reaching that conclusions on the neuropsychological sequelae of cerebrovascular occlusive disease cannot be transferred directly to patients after SAH.

8.2. Strengths and weakness of neuropsychological measures in patients after SAH

Only systematic neuropsychological diagnostics can yield objective information on the factual cognitive functional level of a patient with brain damage. Neuropsychological diagnostics covers a vast multitude of measuring instruments and testing procedures in order to assess the cognitive functional level of patients after brain damage (Lezak, 1983). The selection of the appropriate tests depends on the individual interests and inclinations of the respective researcher or clinician. Therefore, at this point only some general comments on test procedures applied so far in diverse publications and own studies on the neuropsychological sequelae after SAH can be made. A general principle consists in the application of only such standardized and normated test procedures whose validity and reliability for neuropsychological questions has been verified empirically (Lezak, 1983). In the following, Table 1 contains a general listing of the most common and most important neuropsychological abnormalities due to acquired brain damage without already bearing concrete reference to the neuropsychological sequelae of SAH.

Disturbances of learning and memory belong, according to the general opinion, to the most common sequelae of acquired brain damage. This holds especially true for patients after SAH, whose impairments of short-term memory constitute the by far most frequent neuropsychological symptoms (Hütter et al., 1999; Hütter, Gilsbach and Kreitschmann, 1995; Hütter and Gilsbach, 1993; 1992). In connection with the investigation of the neuropsychological sequelae of SAH, the tests should cover before all those areas of cognitive function in which impairments in this patient group can typically be found. These are in detail short- and long-term memory as well as different aspects of attention. Since aphasic language disorders can occur even in neurologically unimpaired patients after SAH, the application of at least an aphasia screening test is called for (Hütter and Gilsbach, 1993).

The use of not normated or unstandardized experimental neuropsychological test procedures is associated with the great difficulty of finding an adequate control group that is superior to a good sample of probands

Table 1. Neuropsychological impairments after acquired brain damage

1. Visual field defects
2. Neglect
3. Defects of visuo-spatial constructive capacities
4. Distortions of face and object recognition
5. Memory disorders
6. Language disturbances (aphasias)
7. Deficits in problem solving
8. Impairments of motor fine coordination
9. Impairments of complex sensori-motor coordination
10. Apraxias
11. Attention deficits
12. Mental rigidity
13. Dementia
14. Deficits of concentration capacity
15. Personality changes/emotional disorders
16. Behavioral disorders

without brain damage, keeping in mind the hypothesis in question. For specific hypotheses, the problem emerges which group of patients with brain damage or which specific comparable group of SAH patients is suitable to answer the question. The question of the individual functional cognitive level of each individual patient (a standard question in everyday neuropsychological diagnostics), can only be answered by an analytic single case approach, in which the test score of the patient is compared to the expected value corrected by age and education that corresponds to the mean value of an appropriate comparative sample according to the test norms (Lezak, 1983). In common practice, a cognitive deficit in neuropsychological diagnostics is then indicated if the test score of the patient lies below two or more standard deviations (SD) of the mean value of the test norms. In test norms that stem from a sample of probands without brain damage, such a score corresponds to a test performance that can be found, depending on the respective test (or the respective distribution of the sample), in approximately 3–4% of the not brain damaged probands in the normal sample. Norms derived of patients with brain damage are subject to the problem that they are based on a "uniformity hypothesis" of the neuropsychological sequelae of brain damage. The underlying "uniformity hypothesis" of homogeneous and unspecific effects of brain damage irrespective of etiology and location can not be maintained at present in this simple form. Also, the comparison of the group means is not practical in patients after SAH. It could be demonstrated in several studies that the group means in nearly all neuropsychological tests in patients after SAH corresponded to the expected value, even if some patients exhibited substantial cognitive deficits (Hütter, Gilsbach and Kreitschmann, 1995; Hütter and Gilsbach, 1993). In the majority of neuropsychological tests, the comparison of group means to a sample of probands without brain damage would, therefore, not yield a statistically significant difference in the group means in patients in the chronic state after SAH and mislead to the erroneous conclusion that these patients are neuropsychologically intact. Furthermore, it should be kept in mind in the compilation of neuropsychological tests for the investigation of patients after SAH that also the consequences of secondary complications, the effects of medical management and especially the effects of surgical procedures and events can be assessed. Therefore, the core of a neuropsychological test battery for the use in SAH patients should comprehend at least tests of short- and long-term memory, functions of attention and an aphasia screening test such as the Token Test. For the investigation of patients in the acute stage of the illness, it is a prerequisite that the selected tests can be applied sensibly in a bed-side testing arrangement (Hütter and Gilsbach, 1996a).

8.2.1. Neuropsychological assessment of frontal brain functions

For theoretical reasons as well as because of the pathology and pathophysiology of SAH, the use of at least one measurement procedure sensitive for fronto-cortical dysfunction is recommended in this patient group. Among neuropsychologists, there exists a long-lasting debate on which test procedures can be regarded as sensitive for fronto-cortical dysfunctions. There is an increasing consent, that fluency tests, tasks according to a Go/NoGo paradigm and the Wisconsin Card Sorting Test (WCST) belong to those standardized and normated measures available at present that can be regarded suitable for such questions (Hütter, 1997b). In the meanwhile, the majority of authors agree on the opinion that conventional intelligence tests are not suited for the diagnostics of frontal cognitive dysfunctions (Walsh, 1987; Stuss and Benson, 1986; Mesulam, 1986; Hecaen and Albert, 1975; Teuber, 1964). The most common tests of frontal brain function are the WCST (Heaton et al., 1993), the Go/NoGo Test (Drewe, 1975), verbal fluency tasks (Benton, 1968) and labyrinth tests (Porteus, 1950). Table 2 gives an overview of test procedures for the investigation of frontal brain function.

The German version of the Stroop Test is also termed color-word-interference test (Farbe-Wort-Interferenztest; FWIT; Bäumler, 1985). According to the developer, this test especially designed for neuropsychological questions measures the strength of controlled information processing in relation to the strength of automatized processing (Bäumler, 1985). By means of the FWIT, three different performance parameters are assessed: 1. susceptibility for interference, 2. selectivity and 3. word finding capacity. The FWIT is regarded as sensitive by the test author for frontal brain damage (Bäumler, 1985). However, several studies exist meanwhile, which question the capability of the Stroop Test for the assessment of fronto-cortical cognitive functional deficits (Hütter, 1997b). The Wisconsin Card Sorting Test (WCST) is a procedure oftentimes made use of for the measurement of frontal brain function. The WCST (Heaton et al., 1993) is a sorting task, in which the proband must discover the sorting principle of

Table 2. Neuropsychological diagnostic procedures of "frontal" brain functions

Standardized tests	Non-standardized tests
Wisconsin Card Sorting Test (WCST)	Tower-of-Hanoi task
Heaton et al. (1993)	Anzai & Simon (1979); Shallice (1982)
Go/NoGo test	Mental Rotation tasks
Drewe (1975)	Shepard & Metzler (1971)
Halstead Categories test	Clinical interviews; proxy ratings
Halstead (1947)	Lezak (1982); Hütter & Gilsbach (1995a;b)
Porteus Labyrinth test	Labyrinth tasks
Porteus (1950)	Walsh (1987); Karnath, Zimmermann & Wallesch (1991)
Benton Word Fluency test	Estimation tasks
Benton (1968)	Smith & Milner (1984)
Stroop test (FWIT)	Behavioral observation
Bäumler (1985)	Luria (1970); Goldberg & Costa (1986)

cards that differ in several dimensions (color, pattern, number of patterns) by trial and error. After ten successive correct answers the sorting principle is changed without prior warning and the proband must deduce the new sorting principle from the answers of the experimenter. Milner (1963) and Robinson et al. (1980) observed that after frontal brain damage, patients were more impaired in the WCST than patients with more posteriorly located lesions. On the other hand, Anderson et al. (1991) found in a well controlled study with relatively exact lesion location in 49 patients with either uni- or bi-lateral frontal brain damage due to vascular disease or an operated tumor (meningeoma or solitary metastasis) no worse test performance in the WCST in comparison to patients with non-frontal brain damage.

A conclusive appraisal of the sensitivity and specificity of the various procedures is at present not possible. However, already the early studies of Drewe (1975;1974) showed that the Go/NoGo Test and the WCST can be regarded as sensitive for the assessment of disturbed frontal brain function. According to the results of a study of Pendleton et al. (1982), the WCST was more sensitive for a frontal lesion than the Categories Test, whereas the latter was more sensitive again than the WCST for a non-frontal brain disturbance. Of all tests, however, the Word Fluency Test (WFT) exhibits the highest sensitivity for organic frontal brain damage (Crockett et al., 1986; Pendleton et al., 1982; Benton, 1968). On the other hand, performance in the WFT is also influenced considerably by lesions of the thalamus, general dementia, subcortical and left-hemispheric damage. In the study by Crockett et al. (1986), the WCST, the WFT and the Categories Test were, therefore, investigated with respect to how well these measures were able to distinguish between psychiatric patients, patients with non-frontal brain damage and those with frontal brain damage. By means of the used test procedures, 66.3% of the patients could be classified correctly into their group. The WFT

Brower, 1987; Mesulam, 1985; Van Zomeren, Brower and Deelman, 1984; Posner and Boies, 1972).

A modern conception of attention stems from Posner and Petersen (1990), who differentiate between three partial aspects of attention, namely selectivity, capacity and controlled processing. In neuropsychology, impairments of attention are commonly differentiated according to these areas and investigated separately. The difficulty exists, however, to assign the respective aspect to the different impairments of performance. Attention must rather be regarded as a basic cognitive function whose disturbance is followed by a multitude of cognitive functional impairments. A minimal neuropsychological assessment of attention should at least include the examination of cognitive speed of processing, selectivity and attention capacity (Hütter, Kreitschmann-Andermahr and Gilsbach, 1998; Hütter and Gilsbach, 1996a). For the diagnostics of functions of attention most of all paper and pencil tests and instrument-based procedures are used, whereby the computer-assisted attention test battery of Zimmermann and Fimm (1992) constitutes a common procedure in Germany for instrument-based attention diagnostics. For the assessment of basic functions of attention oftentimes three different tasks of the computerized neuropsychological test battery of Zimmermann and Fimm (1992) were used in the studies of the research group around the author of this book. Those subtests of the test battery of Zimmermann and Fimm (1992) regularly applied in their own studies served for the evaluation of basic components of attention such as simple reaction time, alertness as the ability to react faster to an expected stimulus, the capacity of divided attention and a visual task according to a Go/NoGo paradigm (Nestor, Parasuraman and Haxby, 1991; Posner and Petersen, 1990; Nebes and Brady, 1989; Grady, Grimes and Petronas, 1989; Posner, 1982; Drewe, 1975). These three tasks are supposed to assess four of the basic functions of attention, postulated by Ben-Yishai, Piasetsky and Rattok (1987) as existing next to vigilance.

Alertness implies the ability to react more quickly to an anticipated stimulus (Zimmermann and Fimm, 1992; Posner and Petersen, 1990; Posner, 1982). This stimulus is announced in random distance but close in time to the critical stimulus by a warning signal, save that a set time distance can be anticipated between both stimuli. The alertness test examines the ability for the phasic elevation of the level of attention according to the theory of Posner and Rafal (1987) and of Posner and Boies (1972). The investigation of divided attention consists in the simultaneous pursuit of two quickly presented tasks in different sensory modalities, the requirement being a discovery of the critical stimulus as fast as possible (Nestor, Parasuraman and Haxby, 1991; Posner and Petersen, 1990; Nebes and Brady, 1989; Grady, Grimes and Petronas, 1989; Posner, 1982). In the task "divided attention" out of the test battery of Zimmermann and Fimm (1992), the attention capacity in the sense of Kahnemann (1973) is measured by means of a simultaneous optical and auditory task. The Go/NoGo task assesses the ability to react selectively to critical stimuli and to ignore other physically similar stimuli (Drewe, 1975). Hereby, the strength of the perseveration tendency is registered which is inversely proportional to the strength of the tendency to interrupt an automatic train of action intentionally. A lack of selectivity which is expressed in perseverative and repetitive behavior was observed in patients with frontal brain damage but also after damage of other brain regions (Goldberg and Bilder, 1987; Canavan, Janota and Schurr, 1985; Drewe, 1975; 1974; Allison and Hurwitz, 1967). In so far Go/NoGo tasks can also be regarded as indicators for the performance capacity of fronto-cortical areas (Hütter, 1997b).

The independence of the basic components of attention of each other is indicated by the investigation of Ben-Yishai, Piasetsky and Rattok (1987), in which no generalization of the effect of neuropsychological rehabilitation from one aspect of attention to another was shown. In a study by Hütter and Gilsbach (1996a), 28 patients in a median of 5 days after early surgery on a ruptured intracranial aneurysm completed tasks for the evaluation of simple reaction time, alertness and divided attention capacity next to neuropsychological tests. No significant common variance was found between simple reaction time and (phasic) alertness ($r = 0.06$; $p > 0.05$). Furthermore, no association emerged between the investigated functions of attention and different aspects of concentration capacity, as measured by means of the test d2 ($r = 0.02$ up to $r = 0.32$; $p > 0.05$), nor between the different functions of attention investigated ($r = 0.12$ up to $r = 0.34$; $p > 0.05$). On the one hand, this means that concentration performance is essentially independent of functions of attention. On the other hand, the three components examined in the study of Hütter and Gilsbach (1996a) are not associated substantially with each other, so that they can be regarded as independent aspects of the theoretical construct of attention (Hütter and Gilsbach, 1996a). A theoretically important result of the study of Hütter and Gilsbach (1996a) consists in the finding that simple reaction time and alertness were statistically independent of each other and, therefore, constitute independent components of attention. This should also have consequences for the terminology. In the future, the expression "tonic alertness" for simple reaction time should be abandoned since this suggests an empirically not justified association with (phasic) alertness. The latter should, therefore, in the future be simply called "alertness". Vigilance as the fifth basic function of attention has not been taken into consideration in own studies because it would have elongated the investigation time unjustifiably.

8.2.4. Neuropsychological measurement of aphasic language disorders, complex sensorimotor coordination, concentration capacity, visuoconstructive capacity, abstract thinking and general intelligence

Aphasia is the impairment of the ability to express oneself by means of language as well as to understand spoken words due to damage of the central nervous system. Those two fundamental areas of language competency may be disturbed to a different extent. Aphasias are a major domain of neuropsychological diagnostics and rehabilitation, because the ability to communicate is of utmost importance for all areas of daily life. Therefore, the quality of life of aphasic patients is severely disturbed (Hütter, Engell and Huber, 1995). Most of all mild aphasic disorders can be overlooked even if they lead to a substantial impairment in the daily life of the patients (Hütter, Kreitschmann and Gilsbach, 1995). This implies that a systematical assessment of aphasia is indispensable after brain damage. The Aachen Aphasia Test (AAT) is a standard procedure for the German-speaking population to assess severity, syndrome and specific type of an aphasia (Huber et al., 1983). Next to the relatively lengthy AAT, it is possible to employ the Token Test (Orgass, 1982) for aphasia screening. The Token Test reliably allows the diagnosis and quantification of the severity of an aphasic language disturbance (Orgass, 1982). The Token Test is easy to perform and separates between aphasics and non-aphasics with a high degree of dependability, but does not allow a classification of the aphasic syndrome. During the Token Test, the patient must follow a series of verbal instructions in increasing complexity to complete simple tasks with a batch of plastic tokens of different colors and forms (circles and squares) that come in two different sizes.

The Wiener Determinationsgerät (Klebelsberg, 1960) is a device to test reaction time and the speed of sensorimotor coordination. Additionally, resistance to stress also plays an important role. The patients must react to different tone and light signals with a number of specific movements of the hands and feet (pushing buttons, pressing pedals). The speed of stimulus presentation is independent of the reactions of the probands and increases continuously during the first half of the experiment in order to decrease again in the second half. This testing procedure had initially been developed in order to assess the capacity to drive a car. The test norms based on the data of 600 healthy probands (TÜV Baden, 1976). Three parameters of performance are assessed by means of the Wiener Determinationsgerät: 1. number of correct reactions, 2. absolute number of errors and 3. percentage of errors. This device has been validated and well established for questions of traffic psychology. The Wiener Determinationsgerät is often used in neuropsychological diagnostics, however, a validation for neuropsychological questions is missing as of yet. It is, moreover, subject to the disadvantage that in the scope of neuropsychological diagnostics the number of impaired patients is probably overestimated to due to the high complexity of the task. Although the Wiener Determinationsgerät is a valid instrument for the prognosis of traffic fitness, in the context of neuropsychological questions, its incorporation into theories of cognition psychology or neuropsychology is, however, not given because of the multimodal complexity of the tasks. The paradigm "floats" so to speak over neuropsychologically defined functions and can, therefore, at best only establish a diffuse relationship to defined disturbances of brain function.

Concentration capacity can be measured reliably and with prognostic validity concerning the later ability of the patient to return to work, with the d2 test, the German modification of the Bourdon Wiersma Dot Cancellation Test (Rauchfleisch, 1983; Brickenkamp, 1978). As a paper and pencil test, the d2 requires the marking of as many critical signs "d2" within a time span of 20 seconds. Therefore, the concentration test d2 measures the ability to discriminate under time pressure as many critical signs as possible selectively out of a context of similar signs. This test evaluates four different parameters of concentration capacity. These are 1. total number of correctly marked items, 2. percentage of errors, 3. total performance minus errors, and 4. continuity of performance (Brickenkamp, 1978). It must be made clear, however, that the reliability of the fourth performance parameter is unsatisfactory for neuropsychological questions and should be abandoned in the future (Rauchfleisch, 1983).

The subtest 9 "visuoconstructive capacity" (LPS-RV) of the Leistungsprüfsystem (LPS) by Horn (1983) investigates the ability to imagine geometrical figures three-dimensionally. The task itself consists in counting the number of faces of these figures. The number of correct solutions is used for the calculation of the test score. The subtest 3 "logical thinking" (LPS-LD) of the Leistungsprüfsystem (LPS) by Horn (1983) is a measure to evaluate the capability of abstraction. The task consists in discovering the abstract principle of order of a series of simple geometric figures and to identify the item that does not comply with this principle. Also in this LPS subtest, the number of correct solutions serves to calculate the test score. Both LPS subtests share the disadvantage that, although they are used relatively often in neuropsychological diagnostics in German-speaking countries, they still lack a validation for neuropsychological questions. The WIP (Dahl, 1972) is a modified short version of the Hamburg-Wechsler Intelligence Test for adults (HAWIE). It consists of the four subtests "general knowledge", "picture completion", "mutualities finding" and "mosaic test". The WIP has the advantage of time economic application in comparison to the full HAWIE-version and shares approximately 90% of the variance with the HAWIE-intelligence quotient (Dahl, 1972).

8.3. The measurement of health-related quality of life of patients after SAH by means of the Aachen Life Quality Inventory (ALQI)

8.3.1. The concept of health-related quality of life

In neurosurgery, the overall treatment result of patients after SAH or after traumatic brain injury is generally assessed using the GOS (Jennett and Bond, 1967). For the evaluation of the quality of life of patients with brain tumors, the Karnofsky-Performance Status Scale (Karnofsky and Burchenal, 1949) is frequently employed. There is substantial doubt, however, if such simple scales are at all suitable for measuring the complex construct of quality of life, since they are reduced to the pure physical functional level (Hütter, Gilsbach and Kreitschmann, 1995; Hütter and Gilsbach, 1996b; 1995b; 1993; Hütter, 1990; Feinstein, Josephy and Wells, 1986; Yates,

Chalmer and McKegney, 1980; Hutchinson et al., 1979). Next to exclusively organic criteria such as morbidity, mortality, survival time and the purely physical level of function, quality of life of the afflicted patients is increasingly employed as a criterion for the assessment of the psychosocial effects of bodily diseases and the effectiveness of their treatment (Bullinger, 1997; Bullinger, Ludwig and von Steinbüchel, 1991; Hütter, 1990; Aaronson, 1988; Ware, 1984). This led to the consequence that the World Health Organization (WHO) added quality of life with equal impact as a so-called "soft" criterion of therapeutic efficiency to the so-called "hard" criteria for the evaluation of the success of medical therapies (Aboderin and Venables, 1996). The term quality of life originates from politics or the political science, respectively, but was taken up quickly by the social sciences (Viefhues, 1991; Flanagan, 1982; 1975). It lies close at hand, however, that every field of application such as political sciences, sociology or medicine requires a specific conceptualization of life quality (Bullinger, 1997; Hütter and Gilsbach, 1996b; 1995b; Bullinger, Ludwig and von Steinbüchel, 1991; Viefhues, 1991). This also implies that for every area of application a specific operationalization must be developed, since different aspects of quality of life are relevant for each field.

For a long time, a concept of quality of life dominated in medicine that was reduced to the pure physical functional level (Viefhues, 1991; Ware, 1984; Flanagan, 1982; 1975). More recently, a broader conceptualization has gained general acceptance, which led to the adoption of the term of HRQOL (Aaronson, 1988; VanDam and Aaronson, 1988; Ware, 1984). Meanwhile, there is general acceptance on the essential elements of this term (Bullinger, 1997; Aaronson, 1988; VanDam and Aaronson, 1988; Schwarz et al., 1995; 1990; Viefhues, 1991; Ware, 1984). According to this, health-related quality of life (HRQOL) is regarded as a multi-dimensional construct that comprises essentially the areas 1. functional state, 2. illness-related symptoms, 3. psychological and 4. social functioning (Aaronson, 1988). The domain of the functional state hereby comprises the aspects of self-sufficiency, mobility, physical activities and compliance to role models. Even if a far-reaching agreement on definition and content of HRQOL meanwhile exists, concepts of quality of life as applied to bodily ill patients cannot easily be referred to patients with brain damage. Rather, independent, or at least modified conceptualizations adjusted to this patient group are necessary (Hütter, 1997a;b; Hütter and Gilsbach, 1996b; 1995b; Hütter, Gilsbach and Kreitschmann, 1995; Hütter, 1990; Temkin et al., 1989).

8.3.2. Requirements for the investigation of health-related quality of life in patients with brain damage

For the use in patients with brain damage, all procedures for the assessment of life quality available up to now had the disadvantage that specific areas of problems such as cognitive impairments, which should be of considerable importance for this patient group, were not covered. On the other hand,

Table 3. Requirements for a measure of HRQOL in patients with brain damage

1. Complete operationalisation of the construct of health-related quality of life (HRQOL)
2. Good methodological properties in respect to validity, sensitivity and reliability
3. International comparability of results
4. Comparability with the results of studies about HRQOL in other patient groups
5. Complaints and impairments typical of patients with brain damage are covered
6. For methodological reasons focus of items on observable behavior or real situations in daily life which can be objectified
7. Simple response scale in order not to overload the cognitive and decision capacities of the patients
8. Availability of a parallel version for proxy-rating
9. Inclusion not only of the objective functional impairment but also of the subjective impact

rating scales or questionnaires for the evaluation of everyday symptoms of cognitive impairments of function as the Neuropsychological Impairment Scale (O'Donnell et al., 1984a;b) or the Neurobehavioral Assessment Scale (Chernik et al., 1992) simply do not contain all fundamental dimensions of HRQOL regarded as relevant. In sum, these deliberations give rise to a number of prerequisites that must be fulfilled by a method for the evaluation of HRQOL in patients with brain damage (Table 3).

The Helsingborg Declaration on Stroke Management in which the routine assessment of HRQOL of stroke patients is called for also speaks for the increasing importance of the concept of health-related life quality in patients with brain damage. Furthermore, quality of life is declared a mandatory variable for clinical research and a treatment goal pertaining to quality of life in patients is defined for the year 2005 (Aboderin and Venables, 1996). For the research area of quality of life in patients with brain damage, meanwhile the first research experiences on the application and methodological suitability of different standard procedures in stroke patients exist (Anderson, Laubscher and Burns, 1996; Dorman et al., 1996; Visser et al., 1996; Hütter, Engell and Huber, 1995; Ebrahim, Barer and Nouri, 1986). Table 4 lists the respective procedures.

Due to the great difference to patients after cerebrovascular occlusive disease, these results cannot be transferred readily to patients after SAH. Moreover, there are advanced methodological and conceptual efforts to

Table 4. Measures for the assessment of HRQOL, whose methodological properties have been already examined or are under examination

1. Medical Outcome Study (MOS) short form 36 (SF 36); Anderson, Laubscher and Burns (1996)
2. EORTC EuroQuol (QLCQ-30); Dorman et al. (1996)
3. Nottingham Health Profile; Ebrahim, Barer and Nouri (1986)
4. Aachen Life Quality Inventory for Aphasics (ALQI-A); Hütter, Engell and Huber (1995)
5. Sickness Impact Profile (SIP); Visser et al. (1996)
6. Sickness Impact Profile (German version); Hütter and Würtemberger (1997a;b)

examine the quality of life also of patients with epilepsy (Vickrey et al., 1993; Thorbecke, 1994). In 1992, 50 (62%) of 81 centers in the USA performing epilepsy surgery routinely assessed the quality of life of their patients with standardized methods (Vickrey et al., 1993). It is, therefore, sensible to consider these experiences for the development of a measure for the evaluation of HRQOL in patients with brain damage.

8.3.3. Development and methodological qualities of the Aachen Life Quality Inventory (ALQI) for patients with brain damage

The Aachen Quality of Life Inventory (ALQI) is a questionnaire for the assessment of HRQOL in patients with brain damage. The German version of the Sickness Impact Profile (SIP) served as the basis for the development of the ALQI (Hütter and Würtemberger, 1997a;b; Hütter, 1990; Bergner et al., 1981). In the USA, the SIP is a frequently used and methodologically extensively validated questionnaire for the assessment of HRQOL, whose items are formulated on an objectifiable concrete behavioral level (Bergner et al., 1981). Moreover, some experience with the use of the SIP in patients with traumatic brain damage exists (Stambrook et al., 1991; Temkin et al., 1989; Klonoff, Snow and Costa, 1986). The ALQI contains 11 subscales with 10 items each, assessing the following areas of quality of life: 1. “Activation”; 2. “Mobility”; 3. “House-work”; 4. “Social contacts”; 5. “Family relations”; 6. “Ambulation”; 7. “Work”; 8. “Freetime activities”; 9. “Autonomy”; 10. “Communication”; 11. “Cognitive capacity”. As in the SIP, sum scores of total impairment (ALQI Total Score), psycho-social impairment (ALQI Psycho-Social Score) and physical functioning (ALQI Physical Score) can be calculated (Hütter and Gilsbach, 1996b;1995b). Furthermore, a parallel version of the ALQI for proxy-rating of the patient by the life-companion or another relative was developed (Hütter and Gilsbach, 1996b). This was done to account for the problem of decreased introspection in some patients with brain damage. On the other hand, some patients are no longer able to fill in the questionnaire by themselves due to the severity of their impairments (Hütter and Gilsbach, 1995a; McGlynn and Shacter, 1989; Chelune, Heaton and Lehman, 1986). A version of the ALQI based on pictograms for the assessment of quality of life of patients with aphasias has also been developed (Hütter, Engell and Huber, 1995).

A first evaluation of the methodological properties of the ALQI was conducted using a sample of 231 neurosurgical patients with brain damage of different etiology (Hütter and Gilsbach, 1996b; 1995b). Patient age ranged between 16 and 68 years. 146 of the patients investigated had sustained SAH one to five years ago. 51 patients were investigated one to five years after traumatic brain injury and 34 patients approximately one week before surgery on a benign brain tumor. The validity of the proxy-version of the ALQI was assessed on the basis of the data of 163 life-companions of these patients. Table 5 gives an overview of the internal consistency (Cronbach’s Alpha) and the split-half reliability of the self- and proxy-version of the ALQI.

Table 5. Internal consistency of the self- and the proxy-rating version of the Aachen Life Quality Inventory (ALQI)

		ALQI self-rating version		ALQI proxy-rating version	
ALQI subscales	No. items	Cronbach's Alpha[1]	Split-half Guttman[2]	Cronbach's Alpha[1]	Split-half Guttman[2]
Activation	10	0,85	0,82	0,83	0,84
Mobility	10	0,86	0,84	0,88	0,83
House-work	10	0,88	0,90	0,90	0,92
Social contact	10	0,80	0,83	0,84	0,85
Family relations	10	0,74	0,70	0,78	0,78
Ambulation	10	0,81	0,87	0,78	0,82
Work	10	0,71	0,73	0,77	0,77
Free-time activities	10	0,89	0,85	0,86	0,82
Autonomy	10	0,68	0,69	0,88	0,88
Communication	10	0,78	0,71	0,84	0,80
Cognition	17	0,91	0,92	0,92	0,92
Psycho-social score[3,4]	50	0,94	0,87	0,94	0,89
Physical score[3,4]	40	0,93	0,81	0,94	0,77
Total score[3,4]	107	0,97	0,92	0,97	0,92

[1]Cronbach's Alpha coefficient for internal consistency
[2]Guttman's split-half reliability
[3]Without the subscale "Work"
[4]Without the items about the social status and the single items about illness complaints

For both ALQI versions, the degree of internal consistency can be regarded as excellent to satisfactory for the sum scores as well as for the individual subscales. The validity of the two ALQI versions was verified by means of Spearman rank-order correlations and a number of clinical ratings with known prognostic significance. Table 6 gives an overview of the respective correlations with the ALQI subscales as well as the sum scores of the self- and proxy-rating.

As can be seen from Table 6, a large number of significant but moderate correlations emerged. Table 7 provides a survey of associations between the ALQI sum scores and a broad spectrum of neuropsychological tests of function in a group of $n = 51$ patients one to five years after traumatic brain injury.

Apart from the complex relationship existing between subjective complaints in daily life and cognitive capacity measured by neuropsychological tests, the results can be regarded as an important illustration of the validity of both ALQI versions. A correlation of 0.81 ($n = 163$) emerged between the self- and proxy-rating version of the ALQI, which can be regarded as sufficient for the assumption of parallelism of both instruments. This holds especially true for the specific conditions relevant for the relationship between self- and proxy-rating in patients with brain damage (Hütter and Gilsbach, 1995a).

Table 6. Validity of the self- and proxy-rating version of the ALQI

	ALQI self-rating version			ALQI proxy rating version		
External criteria	ALQI Total Score	ALQI Physical Score	ALQI Social Score	ALQI Total Score	ALQI Physical Score	ALQI Social Score
Rating according to the GOS (n = 231)	0,32*	0,37**	0,27**	0,32**	0,39**	0,25**
Rating according to Hunt & Hess (n = 146)	0,24*	0,18*	0,23*	0,28**	0,26*	0,23*
Severity of the bleeding Fisher Score (n = 146)	0,15*	0,14	0,13	0,20*	0,21*	0,18*
Duration of coma in days (n = 43)[1]	0,33*	0,39*	0,25	0,12	0,16	0,06
Glasgow Coma Score (n = 22)[1]	0,07	−0,16	0,17	0,22	−0,17	0,30*
Aachen Coma Score (n = 51)[1]	−0,32*	−0,31*	−0,28	−0,21	−0,32*	−0,28

*p < 0,01; **p < 0,001
[1]Pearson correlation coefficient

8.4. Disturbances of affectivity and personality in patients after brain damage

For a long time emotional and motivational aspects of brain damage have been neglected in neuropsychological research (Thompson, 1988; Prigatano, 1986; Simonov, 1986). On the other hand, changes of personality and emotional disturbances belong to the generally accepted sequelae of brain damage. In spite of increasing research activities, hitherto concepts on changes of personality and emotional disturbances after brain damage remain controversial up to the present day (Hütter and Gilsbach, 1995a). Luria (1969) expressed the opinion that personality changes after brain damage result of disturbances of concentration, attention and the impairment of the ability to carry out tasks that require complex sequences of mental activity. Insofar, Luria (1969) ascribed personality and affective changes to impairments of the cognitive system. The majority of studies on the relationship between changes of personality and affectivity and acquired brain damage is concerned with the consequences of frontal brain damage. The psychological sequelae of brain damage of other location has been investigated far less frequently.

In a comprehensive review on emotional changes in patients with prefrontal lesions, Fuster (1989) identified apathy and emotional indifference as a constant sequel that was independent from cognitive impairments. A still powerful assignment of lesions of frontal structures to distinct behavioral disturbances stems from Blumer and Benson (1975). The authors differentiated between two qualitatively totally different personality disorders that

Table 7. Validity of the self- and proxy-rating version of the ALQI-correlations with neuropsychological tests (n = 51)

	ALQI self-rating version			ALQI proxy-rating version		
Neuropsychological function[1]	ALQI Total Score	ALQI Physical Score	ALQI Social Score	ALQI Total Score	ALQI Physical Score	ALQI Social Score
Aphasia Token Test#	0,29*	0,14	0,34*	0,36*	0,23	0,42*
Figural short-term memory	0,06	0,09	0,04	−0,12	−0,20	0,06
Verbal short-term memory	−0,32*	−0,20	−0,33*	−0,34*	−0,28	−0,35*
Figural long-term memory	−0,40*	−0,34*	−0,38*	−0,37*	−0,34*	−0,34*
Verbal long-term memory	−0,12	−0,15	−0,07	−0,09	−0,22	−0,01
Concentration/ speed	−0,33*	−0,29*	−0,29*	−0,45*	−0,45*	−0,41*
Concentration/ accuracy	−0,12	−0,18	−0,08	−0,13	−0,22	−0,07
Concentration error-reduced	0,32*	−0,27	−0,28	−0,42*	−0,41*	−0,39*
Simple reaction time (msec)#	0,34*	0,22	0,34*	0,38*	0,37*	0,37*
Alertness	0,00	0,01	0,00	0,00	0,01	0,00
Divided attention reaction time (msec)#	0,27	0,18	0,29	0,34*	0,35*	0,32*
Divided attention omissions#	0,12	0,18	0,10	0,27	0,37*	0,18
Go/NoGo task reaction time (msec)#	0,34*	0,32*	0,30*	0,38*	0,49**	0,30*
Go/NoGo task errors#	0,30*	0,40**	0,20	0,32*	0,47**	0,20

*p < 0,01; **p < 0,001
[1]Pearson correlations
#Raw scores

resulted of damage to different frontal regions. The first type results of damage to the dorso-lateral convexity and is distinguished by apathy, lack of initiative, the inability to plan in advance, loss of emotional resilience and indifference. In this state, the patients seem depressive, which is, however, not supposed to correspond to a "true" depression. For this reason, Blumer and Benson (1975) introduced the term "pseudo-depression". The second type is the consequence of fronto-orbital lesions and demonstrates a childish-egoistic behavior, garishness, combined with sexually tinted inadequate humor (Blumer and Benson, 1975). This type was called "pseudo-psychopathic" by the authors. It is remarkable that the authors' own cases on whom Blumer and Benson (1975) founded their theory all exhibited a bifrontal lesion. According to Blumer and Benson (1975), these changes should basically be observed also after unilateral frontal damage. The question remains, however, in how far already unilateral lesions of frontal brain areas lead to personality changes (Benton, 1968).

Stuss and Benson (1984) implicitly performed a differentiation of psychological symptomatology after frontal brain damage into two variants, and attributed disinhibited and tactless behavior, garishness, emotional lability, carelessness, boasting, euphoria and childish-egoistic behavior to the first. In the second variant, apathy, lethargy, indifference also with regard to the own deficits, sluggish thinking, neglect of the own appearance and insatiable eating were to be found (Stuss and Benson, 1984). Thompson (1988) observed, that due to a frontal lesion, emotional changes such as in- or decrease of fear, depression or euphoria could be the immediate consequence. Robinson et al. (1984) found in stroke patients with left-sided anterior lesions significantly more severe depressiveness as opposed to other localizations. On the other hand, Dam, Petersen and Ahlgren (1989) reported exactly the opposite finding, that much more right-hemispheric in comparison to left-frontal lesions were associated with increased depressiveness. House et al. (1990) and Sinyor et al. (1986) did not find any association at all between frontal lesion location and depression. In a study by Hütter and Gilsbach (1995a), patients after SAH who exhibited frontal infarctions on CCT presented with significantly lower depression scores. Moreover, Hütter and Gilsbach (1995a) found, that patients with frontal infarcts cared significantly less about their state of health, although they rated themselves subjectively just as impaired as all other patients and presented with the same degree of objectifiable neuropsychological deficits.

8.4.1. Psychopathological measures

Psychopathological diagnostics of patients with brain damage predominantly aims at those disorders of emotional adjustment, personal experience, behavior and personality that can occur in the wake of acquired brain damage. Here, the problem exists that it is very difficult to differentiate between the direct consequences of organic brain damage and the reactions of the patients to their illness such as emotional reactions or effects of illness coping. Furthermore, all measures of psychopathological diagnostics have been developed for the use in patients without brain damage. It remains, therefore, questionable in how far the assumptions associated with the respective measures and methodological standards can also be applied to patients with brain damage. A number of procedures for the assessment of depressiveness is consequently subject to the problem that some neurological symptoms of the illness may lead to falsely positive answers to some of the items and, therefore, to exaggerated depression scores (Arnold and Pössl, 1995). The emotional adjustment of patients after SAH is probably also influenced by the psychic reactions to the trauma of the bleeding and

Table 8. Psychopathological syndromes following acquired brain damage

1. Organic personality disorder
2. Apathy and loss of interests
3. Impairment of social judgement
4. Aggressiveness or rage
5. Affective lability
6. Organic affective syndrome (e.g. depression)
7. Organic psychosocial maladjustment
8. Frontal lobe syndrome

the subjective fear of a renewed SAH (Hütter, 1998). Table 8 lists the most frequent psychopathological syndromes related to acquired brain damage.

Next to the application of standardized procedures, the interpretation of which should consider the above mentioned problems, it is recommended for the diagnostics of brain organic psychopathological changes to also question the life-partners and next of kin of the patients about possible changes (Hütter and Gilsbach, 1995a).

8.5. The assessment of psychological adjustment after SAH by means of the revised Freiburger Personality Inventory (FPI-R)

8.5.1. The FPI-R – a brief outline

The Freiburger Personality Inventory in its revised form (FPI-R) is a self-assessment questionnaire for the evaluation of psychological adjustment, consisting of 138 items and containing the following 12 bipolar subscales: 1. "Life-satisfaction versus dissatisfaction", 2. "Social orientation versus selfishness", 3. "Ambition versus low ambition", 4. "Self-consciousness versus self-assurance", 5. "Irritability versus calm", 6. "Aggressiveness versus low aggressiveness", 7. "Strain versus low strain", 8. "Bodily complaints versus no bodily complaints", 9. "Health concerns versus no concerns about the own health", 10. "Openness versus social desirability", 11. "Extroversion versus introversion", 12. "Emotional lability versus emotional stability" (Fahrenberg, Hampel and Selg, 1985; 1984). The norms of the FPI-R were determined using a representative sample of the general population consisting of N = 2035 persons (n = 952 men and n = 1083 women) with an age between 16 to 85 years. Values of three or more stanine scores beyond the mean, corresponding to a deviation of two standard deviations (SD) can be regarded as significant disturbances of psychological adjustment. Such a value corresponds to a score occurring in one extreme direction in 4% of the probands in the normative sample of the FPI-R (Fahrenberg, Hampel and Selg, 1985; 1984). In several studies, different aspects of the validity and specificity of the FPI-R could be demonstrated empirically (Pfingstmann and Baumann, 1986; Krampen, 1986; Schmidt and König, 1986; Schmidt, Häcker and Schwenkmetzger, 1985; Fahrenberg,

Hampel and Selg, 1985; 1984). The FPI-R was protected against possible confounding effects of different answer tendencies in order to minimize the bias resulting of the self-report methodology (Borkenau and Amelang, 1986; Fahrenberg, Hampel and Selg, 1985). For this reason, a control scale was integrated into the FPI-R for the identification of such probands habitually tending to answer in the sense of social desirability (Borkenau and Amelang, 1986; Fahrenberg, Hampel and Selg, 1985).

8.5.2. The validity of the FPI-R in patients after SAH

The FPI-R is a meticulously constructed and empirically carefully protected questionnaire method for the assessment of psychological adjustment in the general population without brain damage (Schmidt and König, 1986; Fahrenberg, Hampel and Selg, 1985; 1984; Amelang and Borkenau, 1982). However, it cannot be presumed without doubt that the goodness criteria of the FPI-R also hold true in patients with brain damage in general and especially in patients after SAH. Therefore, before the diagnostic use of the FPI-R in patients after SAH, the applicability of this questionnaire must be investigated separately. Apart from gross disturbances of the introspective capacity, which are, however, rare in patients after SAH (Hütter and Gilsbach, 1995a), it cannot be taken for granted that the validity of the FPI-R subscales is also given in this patient group. A restriction of the power of the FPI-R in patients after SAH consists most of all therein, that it is at least questionable if and in how far certain emotional disturbances of SAH patients such as the often described emotional impulsiveness can be apprehended. However, a number of empirical findings support the validity of the FPI-R also in this special patient group (Hütter, 1998; Hütter, Gilsbach and Kreitschmann, 1995).

The data of 58 patients in the chronic state after SAH served for the investigation of this question (Hütter, Gilsbach and Kreitschmann, 1995). The apprehended degree of diminished ambition assessed by the respective FPI-R subscale was associated substantially with a perceived lesser performance capacity ($r = 0.46$; $p < 0.01$), reduced motivation ($r = 0.46$; $p < 0.01$) and compromised freetime activities ($r = 0.42$; $p < 0.01$), as assessed by means of a self-report questionnaire (Hütter, Gilsbach and Kreitschmann, 1995). The number of errors in an aphasia screening test (Token Test) correlated significantly ($r = 0.40$; $p < 0.02$) with the degree of bodily complaints (FPI-subscale). The subjective impact of increased headache since the hemorrhage showed substantial correlations with decreased life-satisfaction ($r = -0.42$; $p < 0.01$), increased bodily complaints ($r = 0.71$; $p < 0.001$) and elevated emotional lability ($r = 0.46$; $p < 0.01$), as assessed by the respective FPI-R subscales (Hütter, Gilsbach and Kreitschmann, 1995). Further data analyses were carried out in order to verify the convergent validity of the FPI-R also in patients after SAH (Hütter, 1998). The FPI-R subscales were correlated in patients after SAH with the degree of depressiveness measured by means of the depression inventory of

Beck (BDI) (Hautzinger, 1981; Beck et al., 1961). Statistically significant correlations were found between the degree of depressiveness (BDI) and diminished life-satisfaction ($r = -0.40$; $p < 0.05$), elevated social insecurity ($r = 0.37$; $p < 0.05$) and irritability ($r = 0.34$; $p < 0.05$) as well as increased bodily complaints ($r = 0.39$; $p < 0.05$), measured by the respective FPI-R subscales. Moreover, a highly significant association between the BDI depression score and the FPI-R subscale "emotional lability" with a size of $r = 0.60$ ($p < 0.001$) emerged (Hütter, 1998). These results support the hypothesis of an at least acceptable validity of the FPI-R also in patients after SAH. Nevertheless, it cannot be assumed without restrictions that the FPI-R apprehends psychological disturbances specific for patients after SAH. Thus, the FPI-R is probably not sensitive enough for the tactless and impulsive-uninhibited behavior observed in some patients after SAH which is not addressed sufficiently by the questionnaire.

9. The pattern of cognitive deficits in the chronic state after subarachnoid hemorrhage

9.1. Impact on general intellligence

In connection with the first attempts to exclude an intracranial aneurysm from circulation, already Goldflam (1923) found that SAH leads to specific neuropsychological and psychopathological symptoms, but not to an impairment of general intelligence. A report from Logue et al. (1968) stems from the early days of aneurysm surgery, even before the introduction of the operating microscope and modern intensive care management. Despite the oftentimes drastic consequences of surgery and the untreatable secondary complications, the authors found a normal level of intelligence in the surviving patients. Also in many later studies, substantial cognitive deficits in patients after SAH were found, but in all studies the average intelligence quotient (IQ) was in the normal range (Hütter, Gilsbach and Kreitschmann, 1995; Hütter and Gilsbach, 1993; Säveland et al., 1992; 1986; Ljunggren et al., 1985; Auer, Gallhofer and Auer, 1985; Sengupta, Chinu and Brierley, 1975). In a follow-up study by Sengupta, Chinu and Brierley (1975), as well as in a study by Auer, Gallhofer and Auer (1985), unremarkable IQ mean values were found in the Wechsler Intelligence Test in patients after aneurysm rupture. On the other hand, a large number of patients in both samples complained of decreased general performance capacity, increased irritability and a substantial loss of initiative.

Based on such results, the question arose in how far the subjective complaints of SAH patients could be objectified by means of neuropsychological tests. Auer, Gallhofer and Auer (1985) speculated that the reason for these abnormalities were to be found in the "syndrome of the trephinated patient" in whom exclusively the knowledge to have been operated upon the brain led to the worry to be "off the top". In a study by Hütter and Gilsbach (1993) with 31 patients after early surgery and exclusively good neurological results (GOS = I), neither in the subtests "general knowledge", "picture completion", "mutualities finding" and "mosaic test" of the short version WIP (Dahl, 1972) of the Hamburg Wechsler Intelligence Test, nor in the total IQ of the WIP significant performance deficits were found. In a study by Stenhouse et al. (1991), in 27 patients 12 to 84 months after the rupture and surgical repair of an ACoA aneurysm, the mean value of the Wechsler IQ of 107 (SD 11) was in the normal range. No difference in the IQ mean value was found between neuropsychologically substantially impaired and unimpaired patients (Stenhouse et al., 1991). Also in the sample of Ogden, Mee and

Henning (1993a), the average IQ was in the normal range. These results show that in SAH patients the IQ is mostly independent of the true extent of neuropsychological impairments. Furthermore, it can be concluded from these results that intelligence tests are not suitable for the diagnostics of cognitive deficits in patients after SAH.

9.2. Cognitive deficits after SAH

Depending on the respective cognitive function and the neurological result, the majority of patients after SAH exhibit persisting deficits in individual areas of mental performance. Tidswell et al. (1995) found in 37 patients 6 months and longer after the rupture of an intracranial aneurysm that 65% exhibited a cognitive deficit, at least in one area. In a prospective study, McKenna et al. (1989a) investigated 100 patients three months and one year after aneurysm rupture and late surgery. According to their opinion, the authors could neither find significant cognitive impairments nor restrictions in the daily life of their patients. Nonetheless, in the study of McKenna et al. (1989a), 14% of the neurologically intact patients exhibited two or more cognitive deficits whereas 95% of the neurologically abnormal patients were neuropsychologically impaired. After a conversion of the test scores that is difficult to follow, McKenna et al. (1989a) found no significant difference between SAH patients and a control group of patients after a heart attack. Comparisons of group means are problematical, however, since samples of patients after SAH usually exhibit normal group means in most neuropsychological tests (Hütter and Gilsbach, 1993; Hütter, Gilsbach and Kreitschmann, 1995). Apart from the conversion procedure of the test scores, the power of the results of McKenna et al. (1989a) is additionally restricted by the fact that the used test battery only exhibits a limited sensitivity for SAH patients, since most of all tests of intelligence or tests derived thereof were used. Even in the case of considerable cognitive impairments, SAH patients still perform normally in an intelligence test (Hütter, Gilsbach and Kreitschmann, 1995; Hütter and Gilsbach, 1993; Ogden, Mee and Henning, 1993a; Stenhouse et al., 1991; Säveland et al., 1992; 1986; Ljunggren et al., 1985; Auer, Gallhofer and Auer, 1985; Sengupta, Chinu and Brierley, 1975). Richardson (1991) found deficits of verbal and non-verbal fluency and object-naming next to memory impairments six months after aneurysm rupture. Before all, deficits in fluency tests, as reported by Richardson (1991) point to a persisting impairment of fronto-cortical functions after aneurysm rupture (Hütter, 1997b).

In 81 patients three months after aneurysm rupture, Mercier et al. (1991) found deficits in orientation to space and time and in 9 (11%) patients an aphasic language disturbance. Maier-Hauff, Djoucharda and Hättig (1991) investigated 30 patients between 7 and 42 months after aneurysm surgery. In comparison to a control group of patients without brain damage, aneurysm patients exhibited a significantly worse memory performance and a gradual slowing of reaction time in some of the subtests of the Zimmermann attention test battery. In the study of Ogden, Mee and Henning (1993a), most often impairments in the Trail-Making Test A were found, in which 76% of the patients showed deficits in the speed of visuo-motor coordination. In a retrospective study, 58 patients were investigated neuropsychologically one to five years after SAH by Hütter, Kreitschmann and Gilsbach (1995). The sample consisted of 38 (65%) early operated patients and 20 (35%) patients after spontaneous non-traumatic SAH without a proven cause of the bleeding. Among the patients with an angiographically proven aneurysm, 18 (31%) had a ruptured ACoA aneurysm. The neurological result (GOS) six months after the bleeding had been assessed as good (GOS = I) in 48 (83%) and as fair (GOS = II) in 10 (17%) patients. In different parameters of a complex choice reaction task (Wiener Determinationsgerät), between 31% and 65% of the patients exhibited significant performance deficits. In six (10%) patients, the Token Test provided evidence for an aphasic language disturbance. Only 9 (15%) patients were neuropsychologically unimpaired and had no single cognitive deficit. On the other hand, the mean values of all neuropsychological tests with the exception of the performance parameters of the complex choice reaction task (Wiener Determinationsgerät) were in the normal range (Hütter, Gilsbach and Kreitschmann, 1995). Table 1 gives a survey of the frequency and pattern of cognitive deficits in the study sample of Hütter, Gilsbach and Kreitschmann (1995).

Also in neurologically intact patients, frequently substantial cognitive deficits can be found. Hütter and Gilsbach (1993) found in 31 exclusively early operated patients with a good neurological result (GOS = I) no single patient with a cognitive deficit in visuoconstructive capacity (LPS-Subtest 9) and in logical thinking (LPS-Subtest 3), as well as in the subtests "selectivity", "susceptibility for interference" or "word finding capacity" of the Stroop-Test (FWIT). On the other hand, in 3 (10%) SAH patients with GOS = I, the Token Test revealed a mild to moderate aphasic language disturbance. In the total number of correctly marked items of the concentration test d2, three (10%) patients were impaired (Hütter and Gilsbach, 1993). The most frequent neuropsychological abnormalities were found with 28–62% in a complex choice reaction task (Wiener Determinationsgerät). Heiskanen and Vilkki (1981) investigated 25 patients neuropsychologically between six months and 11 years after aneurysm rupture and surgical repair. Testing was only performed in those patients who were stricken by the disease in childhood or adolescence. At the time of the bleeding, two patients were three months and four years of age. The psychological investigation revealed a similar pattern of deficits as in those patients who had suffered from SAH in the adult age. The emphasis of impairments was seen in the area of learning and memory as well as in abstraction capacity (Heiskanen and Vilkki, 1981). Neither effects of aneurysm location nor side of the surgical approach were found (Heiskanen and Vilkki, 1981).

The cognitive deficits of patients after SAH are similar to those described after mild closed head injury (Uzell, 1988; Uzell, Langfitt and Dolinskas,

Table 1. Cognitive functions examined, neuropsychological tests used and frequency cognitive deficits

Cognitive function	Neuropsychological test	Cognitive deficits	
		No.	%
General intelligence	Wechsler IQ-test short form (WIP)	0	0
Abstraction capacity	subtest Wechsler IQ-test (WIP)	0	0
General knowledge	subtest Wechsler IQ-test (WIP)	0	0
Pictures completion	subtest Wechsler IQ-test (WIP)	0	0
Visuo-spatial construction	subtest Wechsler IQ-test (WIP)	0	0
Concentration (speed)	concentration test d2	3	10
Concentration (error-percent)	concentration test d2	2	7
Concentration (error-reduced)	concentration test d2	4	13
Aphasia screening	Token Test	3	10
Spatial imagination	Leistungsprüfsystem (LPS-RV)	0	0
Logical thinking	Leistungsprüfsystem (LPS-LD)	0	0
Verbal long-term memory	IST verbal memory subtest	6	21
Figural short-term memory	Benton test	16	53
Interference	Stroop test (FWIT)	0	0
Selective attention	Stroop test (FWIT)	0	0
Word-finding capacity	Stroop test (FWIT)	0	0
Complex choice reaction (errors)	Wiener Determinationsgerät	8	28
Complex choice reaction (error-percent)	Wiener Determinationsgerät	18	62
Complex choice reaction time	Wiener Determinationsgerät	17	59

According to Hütter, Gilsbach and Kreitschmann (1995)

1987; Stuss et al., 1985; Gronwall and Wrigthson, 1974). Also here, attention deficits and deficits of short-term memory dominate, without impairments of general intelligence as measured by IQ tests (Hall and Bornstein, 1991). It is rather unlikely, however, that these similarities are based on a similar pathophysiology or damage to the same neuroanatomical structures. On the other hand, there is the possibility that the patterns of deficits are similar because they result of an unspecific "diffuse" brain damage, since after SAH as well as after traumatic brain injury, lesions seen on CCT only correlate weakly with neurological or neuropsychological abnormalities (Teasdale, 1984). A further less likely alternative is that such a pattern of cognitive disturbances is the unspecific expression of the presence of brain damage irrespective of etiology. An empirical clarification of these questions would require the direct comparison of the cognitive deficits in both patient groups. However, such a comparison has not been performed so far.

Also a comparative investigation of patients after SAH and after surgery for a frontal meningeoma would be worthwhile, since it stands to speculate that both patient groups are subject to diffuse frontal brain damage. In the study of Hütter and Gilsbach (1993), multivariate statistical analyses demonstrated a significant unfavorable effect of the severity of the bleeding as assessed by means of the CCT grading of Fisher, Kistler and Davis (1980). This effect was especially pronounced with respect to sensorimotor coordination and the FWIT subtest for the speed of word finding capacity (Hütter and Gilsbach, 1993). This result was interpreted by the authors as evidence for the damaging effect of the subarachnoid blood on the brain, especially on fronto-basal structures (Hütter and Gilsbach, 1993). Such a conceptualization of the mental performance deficits to be found after SAH raises the question about the type of brain damage as the cause of such functional deficits. Based on the available results on the cognitive deficits after SAH, more likely a diffuse damage of especially the paracisternal gray substance with a fronto-basal emphasis than a focal lesion in dependence of aneurysm location can be postulated (Hughes and Oppenheimer, 1969).

9.2.1. Memory deficits after SAH

In a retrospective study, Larsson et al. (1989) investigated 219 patients two to 14 years after SAH with a number of neuropsychological tests with respect to their performance capacity in working memory and verbal short-term memory. Most frequently, impairments of verbal short-term memory were found in this investigation. Unfortunately, Larsson et al. (1989) only used tests for the assessment of verbal memory. Even if memory deficits after SAH have the tendency to be unspecific of modality, the results of Larsson et al. (1989) would have been easier to interpret if the authors had also used tests for the evaluation of aspects of figural memory. Tessier du Cros and Lhermitte (1984) found in 47% of the ACoA patients memory impairments as the most frequent cognitive deficit, which became manifest in the Rey-Österrieth task.

According to the results of the research group around Hütter et al., short-term memory is most of all impaired in SAH patients (Hütter and Gilsbach, 1996a; 1993; 1992; Hütter, Gilsbach and Kreitschmann, 1995; 1994). In the study of Tidswell et al. (1995) there was no single patient among the patients with memory deficits who only presented with a deficit in the verbal modality, but rather exhibited an additional deficit it at least one further test of a non-verbal memory modality. Deficits of short-term learning and remembering also constituted the most common neuropsychological abnormalities after SAH in a study by Tisdwell et al. (1995). Hütter, Gilsbach and Kreitschmann (1995) most frequently found deficits in figural short-term memory (46%; Benton Test). Verbal long-term memory was impaired in 21% of the patients. In a prospective longitudinal study of SAH patients mostly after aneurysm rupture (of whom all 79 aneurysm patients had been operated upon late), Ogden, Mee and Henning (1993a) found memory deficits as the most frequent neuropsychological impairment in 30–88% at the time of discharge from hospital. At the time of follow-up,

12 months later, still 8–46% of their patients exhibited memory deficits. Also Barbarotto et al. (1989) found in patients with ruptured MCA or PCoA aneurysms, that deficits of short-term memory made up the most common neuropsychological impairment with up to 50%. Richardson (1989) also described deficits of short-term memory as the most frequent problem of patients after aneurysm rupture. Laiacona et al. (1989) reported in 43 patients with ruptured ACoA aneurysms also most often impairments of short-term memory. The authors emphasized that impairments of short-term memory were much more frequent than long-term memory deficits. Of 81 patients three months after aneurysm rupture, Mercier et al. (1991) found in 21 (26%) impairments in short-term memory and in 11 (14%) patients deficits in long-term memory. Overall, memory impairments were the most common neuropsychological deficit with a frequency of 40% (Mercier et al., 1991). Also Larsson et al. (1989) found in a retrospective study with 219 patients between two and 14 years after the rupture of an aneurysm most often impairments of short-term memory.

Despite enormous differences in the neuropsychological test procedures used, the majority of the relevant studies concurs in the finding that short-term memory is more frequently impaired that long-term memory in patients after SAH. Next to damage to fronto-basal structures such as the gyrus rectus (Hütter and Gilsbach, 1996a), the nucleus basalis Meynert (Hussein and Archilli, 1996), or paraventricular structures as the septum in the case of intraventricular hemorrhage (Hütter, Kreitschmann-Andermahr and Gilsbach, 1998), also damage to basal paracisternal structures like the uncus, the gyrus parahippocampalis and the hippocampus could constitute an important prerequisite for the presence of the memory deficits after SAH (see Table 1, chapter 4). This damage leads to a disruption of fronto-temporal fibers and the connections between the frontal cortex, hippocampus and limbic system, respectively.

9.2.2. Morphological correlates of cognitive deficits in patients after SAH

Vilkki et al. (1989) investigated 96 patients one year after aneurysm rupture by a number of neuropsychological tests. At the time of follow-up, in all patients a CCT was performed. Infarcted territories were seen on CCT scan in 55% of the patients and in 22% evidence for diffuse brain damage was found (Vilkki et al., 1989). Patients with left-sided infarctions performed significantly worse in all tests of the verbal memory modality, patients with right-sided infarcts performed significantly worse in all tasks of the figural modality. If frontal infarcts were seen on CCT, memory performance was significantly poorer in the affected patients. Contrary to the expectation of the authors, no worse performance occurred in those tests regarded as sensitive for frontal brain functions. Diffuse brain damage (according to CCT criteria) again was associated with a poorer performance in the Stroop-Test, word fluency tests and abstraction capacity, as well as with impairments of object memory and a poorer digit span (Vilkki et al., 1989). In 20 patients between 3 1/2 and 10 years after early surgery for a ruptured intracranial aneurysm, Romner et al. (1989) carried out a cranial MRI scan and a neuropsychological follow-up. Independent of modality, memory deficits were the most frequent neuropsychological disturbances. Deficits in the WCST as evidence for a fronto-cortical cognitive dysfunction were found in 50% of the patients. Interestingly, a frontal lesion was in 66% of the ACoA patients as frequent as after the rupture of an ICA or MCA aneurysm (66%). No substantial correlation between the severity of neuropsychological impairments and the volume loss of brain substance as measured by MRI was found. Considerable neuropsychological abnormalities were present also in patients without brain damage visible on MRI, whereas on the other side, patients with massive damage to the parenchyma seen on MRI were neuropsychologically intact (Romner et al., 1989). Unfortunately, Romner et al. (1989) did not correlate the location of lesions seen on MRI and specific neuropsychological deficits. In a study by Hardemark et al. (1989) the amount of blood on initial CCT, the initial Hunt and Hess grade as well as the acute concentration of S-100 protein in CSF (which is an indicator for neuronal damage) correlated significantly with the results of a neuropsychological follow-up two years later. A substantial correlation was found between the presence of CCT abnormalities like hypodensities or infarcts, the neurological result (GOS) at the time of discharge as well as the initial Hunt and Hess grade and the initial elevation of the S-100 protein the first 5 to 8 days after the bleeding. However, there was no association with the severity of neuropsychological impairments (Hardemark et al., 1989). Moreover, no correlations were found between morphological abnormalities as seen on late CCT scans and the results of neuropsychological testing. Exclusively the enlargement of the ventricles on late CCT correlated substantially with the results of the neuropsychological investigation (Hardemark et al., 1989). Säveland et al. (1996) investigated the correlations between neuropsychological deficits and abnormalities in regional cerebral blood flow (rCBF) measured by a SPECT in 15 patients six months after aneurysm rupture. Only in five patients an association between the localization between SPECT abnormalities and neuropsychological deficits on the level of a simple differentiation in left- versus right-hemispheric cognitive functions could be established. No correlation at all emerged with the severity of neuropsychological impairments (Säveland et al., 1996). Also two case reports showed that neuropsychologically intact patients exhibited considerable SPECT abnormalities, whereas on the other hand, a cognitively substantially impaired patient had a normal SPECT (Säveland et al., 1996). Also in patients with brain contusions, no consistent or differentiated associations between metabolic abnormalities and cognitive deficits could be demonstrated (Ichise et al., 1994). Therefore, it can be concluded that the neuropsychological significance of metabolic abnormalities is generally overestimated and a new conceptual basis of the relationship between hemodynamics and neuropsychological function, especially in pathological states of the brain, has to be defined.

9.2.3. Comparison of the cognitive deficits in the acute and chronic state after SAH

As a rule, SAH leads to considerable impairments in short-term memory, attention, and less frequently, to aphasic language disorders. General intelligence, as measured by conventional IQ tests remains intact. Moreover, the profile of cognitive deficits in the acute stage after SAH is identical to the one observed several years after the acute event (Hütter and Gilsbach, 1996a; Ogden, Mee and Henning, 1993a; Maurice-Williams, Willison and Hartfield, 1991). Even in the first days after aneurysm surgery, impairments of short- and long-term memory and of attention functions and aphasias prevail (Hütter and Gilsbach, 1996a). Table 2 shows a comparison between the frequency of cognitive deficits as described in a study by Hütter and Gilsbach (1996a) in patients some days after aneurysm surgery and in patients in the chronic state one to five years after SAH (Hütter and Gilsbach, 1993). The neurological result had been rated in both groups as good (GOS = I) according to the GOS at six-month follow-up.

In accordance with the results of Maurice-Williams, Willison and Hartfield (1991), also Hütter and Gilsbach (1996a) found memory and attention problems as the most common cognitive deficits in the first days after aneurysm surgery. In the acute stage after SAH, the profile of cognitive deficits is comparable to the persisting cognitive impairments in the chronic

Table 2. Frequency of cognitive deficits in the acute and in the chronic state after early aneurysm surgery

Cognitive function	Neuropsychological test	1–13 (median 5) days after early surgery (N = 28) cognitive deficits[1]		1–5 (median 3) years after early surgery (N = 31) cognitive deficits[1]	
		No.	%	No.	%
Concentration (speed)	test d2	3	11	3	10
Concentration (accuracy)	test d2	11	39	2	7
Concentration (error-reduced)	test d2	3	11	4	13
Aphasia screening	Token test	9	32	3	10
Verbal long-term memory	IST verbal memory	15	54	6	21
Figural short-term memory	Benton test	20	71	16	53

Deficits in different functions of attention increase are not comparable, because different tests have been used which cannot be compared

[1]A cognitive deficit was defined as a test performance >2 SD below the population mean according to the test norms; the Benton test and the Token Test have individual cut-off values for defining a deficit

state (Hütter and Gilsbach, 1996a; Tidswell et al., 1995; Satzger et al., 1995; Ogden, Mee and Henning, 1993a; Vilkki et al., 1989; Sonesson et al., 1989; 1987; McKenna et al., 1989a;b; Bornstein et al., 1987; Ljunggren et al., 1985). However, the frequency of cognitive deficits in some functions such as aphasia and long-term memory is in part considerably higher in the acute stage (McKenna et al., 1989a;b).

10. Neuropsychological effects of aneurysm location

10.1. Are there specific neurobehavioral sequelae depending on the localization of the ruptured aneurysm?

For quite some time, the question of the existence of neuropsychological sequelae of the rupture of an intracranial aneurysm depending on its location has been discussed controversially among neuropsychologists (Hütter and Gilsbach, 1996a; 1992; DeLuca, 1993; 1992a;b; 1990; Irle et al., 1992a;b; DeLuca and Cicerone, 1991; Richardson, 1991; 1989; DeSantis, 1989; Larsson et al., 1989; Lindquist, 1975; Lindquist and Norlen, 1966). However, scientific interest has been focused mainly on the consequences of ruptured aneurysms of the ACoA. Therefore, only few investigations on the sequelae of ruptured aneurysms of other localization exist so far. Two different lines of thought can be found in the scientific literature on the question of the effects of aneurysm location. Some authors come to the opinion that there are specific neuropsychological consequences depending on aneurysm location (Irle et al., 1992a;b; Larsson et al., 1989; Lindquist, 1975; Lindquist and Norlen, 1966). Others again concur in the opinion that SAH leads to unspecific brain damage, that is for the greater part independent of the localization of the ruptured aneurysm (Hütter and Gilsbach, 1996a; 1992; Hütter, Gilsbach and Kreitschmann, 1995; 1994; DeLuca, 1993; 1992a;b; 1990; Richardson, 1991; 1989; DeLuca and Cicerone, 1991). This view is supported by findings according to which there are no substantial differences between the neuropsychological impairments after aneurysm rupture or after spontaneous non-traumatic SAH without a proven source of the bleeding (Hütter, Kreitschmann-Andermahr and Gilsbach, 1998; Hütter, Gilsbach and Kreitschmann, 1994; Ogden, Levin and Mee, 1990; Sonesson et al., 1989). Moreover, in several studies not even specific neuropsychological effects of the side of the ruptured aneurysm (left versus right) occurred (Maurice-Williams, Willison and Hatfield, 1991; Larsson et al., 1989).

On the other hand, one is prone to expect specific neuropsychological sequelae of different aneurysm locations such as the Babif, the PCoA, the MCA or the ICA, because these are oftentimes associated with complicated bleeding patterns and/or a difficult surgical approach. At present, relevant neuropsychological studies on these aneurysm locations are missing. However, there are some indications for the pronounced neuropsychological deficits after the rupture of aneurysms of the vertebro-basilar circulation. Lunsford, Maroon and Vega (1977) described two cases of global amnesia that occurred in patients after rupture and surgery for an aneurysm of the basilar artery. Also in an older study, Takaku et al. (1979) found, that particularly after the rupture of aneurysms of the vertebro-basilar circulation marked cognitive impairments occurred, including severe memory deficits. In a study by Richardson (1991), the few patients with aneurysms of the vertebro-basilar circulation performed significantly worse in an object naming task as compared to patients with aneurysms of other locations. No remarkable differences were found, however, between the other aneurysm locations (Richardson, 1991). Odgen, Utley and Mee (1997) investigated 127 patients between four and seven years after SAH. The only patient with a retrograde amnesia had a ruptured aneurysm of the vertebro-basilar circulation (Odgen, Utley and Mee, 1997).

The study of Barbarotto et al. (1989) with a follow-up of 27 patients after the rupture and operative repair of an MCA or PCoA aneurysm, respectively, belongs to the few investigations which studied the neuropsychological effects of ruptured aneurysms of other localizations than the ACoA. A left-sided MCA aneurysm was found in 10 patients. Abnormalities on CCT were present in 80% of the patients in the MCA group. Of the patients with left-sided MCA aneurysms, 50% exhibited a deficit in verbal short-term memory, while 28% of the patients with a ruptured right-sided aneurysm had a deficit in a figural short-term memory task. It was conspicuous, however, that deficits in figural modalities were also found in patients with left-sided MCA aneurysms, while respective deficits in verbal tasks also occurred in patients with right-sided MCA aneurysms (Barbarotto et al., 1989). In 41% of the PCoA patients, the CCT scan was abnormal. Between 8–20% of these patients showed deficits in various tasks for the assessment of short-term memory. Deficits in the verbal modality rather occurred in patients with left-sided PCoA aneurysms and in the figural modality in patients with right-sided PCoA aneurysms. Exceptions from the rule were seen, on the other hand, in 8–13% of the patients. The authors concluded from these results that after the rupture of MCA and PCoA aneurysms, impairments of short-term memory belong to the most frequent deficits. Furthermore, Barbarotto et al. (1989) could not identify a specific pattern of cognitive deficits depending on aneurysm location. Moreover, Barbarotto et al. (1989) a gradual relationship between the side of the ruptured aneurysm and the modality in which the respective cognitive deficits occurred. However, with regard to the numerous exceptions, this association was supposed to be only weak.

In a study performed by the author of the present monography, a consecutive series of 45 patients was investigated 4 years after the hemorrhage in terms of their HRQOL using the Aachen Life Quality Inventory (ALQI). In 29 patients the ruptured aneurysm had been surgically excluded from circulation, in 24 of them by early surgery. A further 18 patients had sustained a spontaneous non-traumatic SAH without a proven source of the bleeding. The mean age was 47 years with a range between 30 and 69 years. The sample consisted of 20 men and 25 women. Neither in the self-assessed quality of life nor in the proxy-rating by the patients' life-companions, substantial differences between patients after the rupture and surgical repair of an ACoA aneurysm and the other SAH patients emerged. On the other hand, an analysis of variance with the aneurysm locations ACoA, ICA, MCA and PCoA as factors demonstrated in patients with a ruptured ICA aneurysm a significantly worse self- and proxy-rated life quality in the ALQI subscale "House-work" and in the ALQI summary score "Physical Score" (both $p < 0.05$). This difference could be related to the fact that surgery of this aneurysm location is regarded as technically more difficult. Moreover, due to the anatomical situation, hemorrhage of a ruptured ICA aneurysm carries a high risk of damage to functionally relevant parenchyma.

In numerous studies, no effect of aneurysm location could be ascertained. Heiskanen and Vilkki (1981) found no effect of aneurysm location between 6 months and 11 years after the acute event in 25 patients who had sustained aneurysm rupture at an age between 11 and 19 years. Irle et al. (1992b) compared 30 patients with ruptured aneurysms of different locations, 27 after the rupture of an ACoA aneurysm, and 20 patients after surgery for a near-midline tumor. It was found that the aneurysm patients exhibited significantly more memory deficits than the tumor patients without a proven difference between the aneurysm locations. On the other hand, tumor patients had significantly more attention deficits than the aneurysm patients (Irle et al., 1992b). In a retrospective study, Larsson et al. (1989) investigated 219 patients 2–14 years after SAH with respect to their performance capacity in working memory and verbal short- and long-term memory. Impairments of short-term memory were found most frequently. Neither aneurysm location nor side of the ruptured aneurysm (left versus right) had a substantial influence on test performance (Larsson et al., 1989). Unfortunately, Larsson et al. (1989) only used verbal memory tests. No further cognitive functions were investigated additionally. Finally, the power of the results of Larsson et al. (1989) is also decreased by the fact that most of the patients had been operated upon before the introduction of the operating microscope. Also, no modern intensive care management had been available at the time. Furthermore, data on the number of early operated patients are missing and it seems that in most patients no CCT scans are available. These weaknesses make it, therefore, difficult to interpret the results of the study of Larsson et al. (1989) from a present point of view. Also Maurice-Williams, Willison and Hatfield (1991) searched in vain for an effect of the location of the ruptured aneurysm including side (right versus left) on postoperative neuropsychological test performance.

Neither 10 weeks nor 12 months after aneurysm rupture, Ogden, Mee and Henning (1993a) were able to discover differences between different aneurysm locations in neuropsychological test performance in 79 patients in a prospective longitudinal study. Further evidence for the hypothesis of brain damage independent of the location of a ruptured aneurysm stems from a study using functional imaging. Säveland et al. (1996) investigated the regional cerebral blood flow (rCBF) by means of Technetium 99-m

HMPAO SPECT in a sample of patients six months after surgery for a ruptured intracranial aneurysm. Neither the amount of decrease of the rCBF no raneurysm location showed a systematic correlation to the severity of cognitive deficits or to certain localized cognitive functions (Säveland et al., 1996).

10.2. Disconnection syndromes after aneurysm rupture

In several single case studies, it has been described that independent of location, the rupture of an aneurysm may lead to a disconnection syndrome (Levin et al., 1987; Goldenberg et al., 1985; Beukelman, Flowers and Swanson, 1980; Sweet, 1941). Already in 1941 Sweet reported the case of a ruptured aneurysm of the pericallosal artery, which had led to a disconnection syndrome. During the rupture of an aneurysm of the pericallosal artery, damage to the corpus callosum is not improbable, when, based on the anatomical location of the aneurysm and the direction of the bleeding, hemorrhage into the parenchyma of the corpus callosum occurs. Levin et al. (1987) reported on a patient with a ruptured aneurysm of the pericallosal artery who had been investigated four times neuropsychologically 12, 18, 67 and 169 days after surgery, respectively. Apart from a memory deficit, in the beginning a pronounced disconnection syndrome was present, which persisted over time while the memory deficits of the patient improved considerably. This disconnection syndrome points to massive damage to the corpus callosum as a result of the hemorrhage. Indeed, the initial CCT scan performed on admission of the patient showed hemorrhage into the entire corpus callosum, extending from the genu corporis callosi, the corpus up to the splenium (Levin et al., 1987).

Beukelman, Flowers and Swanson (1980) reported of a patient who had sustained SAH due to the rupture of an ACoA aneurysm. According to the surgical report, during late surgery, small parts of subfrontal cerebral parenchyma, most probably the gyrus rectus, were resected, in order to gain better access to the aneurysm. The aneurysm itself was excluded from circulation by clipping of the ACoA. On the second postoperative day, acute hydrocephalus occurred making shunt insertion necessary. Postoperatively, the patient presented with loss of memory, perception disorders, disorientation and disturbances of the control of left-sided extremities. A CCT performed eight weeks after the intervention showed a hypointense area with a diameter of 1–2 cm between the anterior horns of the lateral ventricles. Extensive neuropsychological investigations were performed 45 days and eight months after surgery. According to Beukelman, Flowers and Swanson (1980), clear signs for a disconnection syndrome were found, apart from amnesia, perception difficulties and decreased initiative. The authors interpreted this finding as an indicator for cerebral disconnection due to the rupture of an ACoA aneurysm. However, the majority of the symptoms described by Beukelmann, Flowers and Swanson (1980) correspond much better to a postoperative ACoA syndrome, which can be explained well in this case with the surgical clipping of the ACoA itself. It cannot be excluded that a disconnection syndrome occurred additionally. This would have been, however, a very rare sequel of the rupture of an ACoA aneurysm. Nevertheless, damage to the corpus callosum due to the hemorrhage or as a result of surgery cannot be ruled out. Here, the anterior part of the callosum or the anterior commissure might have been damaged either directly or as a consequence of damage to the perforating vessels. This is not unlikely during surgery of this kind, performed before the advent of microneurosurgery. The disconnection syndrome might also have resulted from damage to the callosum based on the acute hydrocephalus. Finally, own data (Hütter and Gilsbach, 1996a) suggest that the resection of the gyrus rectus as a whole or in part should have contributed to the symptomatology described by Beukelmann, Flowers and Swanson (1980).

Goldenberg et al. (1985) described a patient who was comatose for one week after rupture and operative treatment of an ACoA aneurysm and afterwards remained in a state characterized by akinetic mutism. A neuropsychological investigation carried out six months later revealed indicators for a disconnection syndrome apart from a severe anterograde amnesia with confabulations, disorientation and a lack of spontaneous activity. Moreover, incontinence was present in the patient. A preoperative CCT scan had shown a massive hemorrhage into the interhemispheric fissure. A further CCT performed six months later revealed infarction of at least the anterior two thirds of the callosum, both cingulate gyri as well as the anterior and medial parts of both frontal lobes. Moreover, the CCT was indicative of the presence of hydrocephalus. In so far, the massive deficits of the patient are not surprising. Although a very unusual course is reported here, this case report illustrates the severity of brain damage that can occur in the wake of SAH and a complicated surgical intervention. On the other hand, it also becomes clear that such single case studies are not suited to develop sensible, scientifically sound hypotheses on the anatomical and pathophysiological basis of the cognitive impairments after SAH. A wealth of possible etiological factors (hemorrhage, surgery, vasospasm, hydrocephalus etc.) can lead numerous patterns of substantial brain damage which can cause in rare cases such drastic and exceptional clinical courses.

10.3. Cognitive deficits after rupture and surgical treatment of an aneurysm of the ACoA

10.3.1. Methodological considerations

Since quite some time, considerable interest in the neurobehavioral sequelae of the rupture and operative treatment of ACoA aneurysms exists, which continues to be present also since the introduction of modern microneurosurgery in the late seventies. One reason for this continuous interest is based on the oftentimes described cognitive and psychoorganic symptoms up to Korsakoff psychosis associated with ACoA aneurysm location in the literature. However, the majority of the respective case reports and group studies originates at a time before the introduction of microneurosurgery. The significance of these studies is limited by a variety of factors:

1. Many have been performed before the introduction of the operating microscope and do not comply with the present standard of surgical techniques. Since pharmacological intensive care management of SAH had also not been developed, it is not clear with respect to the described deficits in how far they are the expression of surgical damage and/or of vasospasm or inadequate management;
2. A further group of publications are case reports or include only arbitrarily selected patient groups and no consecutively treated series of ACoA patients. For this reason, these are studies with a patient selection and not cases which can be regarded as typical for the neuropsychological sequelae of ruptured ACoA aneurysms;
3. In most studies an adequate control group of patients with ruptured aneurysms of other locations is missing.

This is, however, required if specific neuropsychological sequelae of the rupture and surgical repair of ACoA aneurysms are to be demonstrated. This also holds true for all other investigations on the neuropsychological sequelae of ruptured aneurysms at other locations. Moreover, attention should be paid to the fact that also clinically comparable groups are formed in the respective studies. In this respect, especially the neurological state on admission to hospital (Hunt and Hess) and the severity of the bleeding (Fisher-Score) as well as further variables, as disturbances of the circulation of cerebrospinal fluid and the severity of vasospasm must be considered. These variables should be included to achieve a minimal standard of patient documentation.

10.3.2. Single case and small group studies

Okawa et al. (1980) found in a sample of 85 ACoA patients, that 66% presented at least with a temporary postoperative amnestic syndrome and considerable changes of personality. These impairments could be observed in 16% of the patients also at the time of long-term follow-up two to three years later (Okawa et al., 1980). Gade (1982) reported that 30% of 48 ACoA patients three months after surgery exhibited a memory deficit with or without Korsakoff syndrome. At a later follow-up, these patients showed no improvement of their symptomatology. On the other hand, Tessier du Cros and Lhermitte (1984) found in 32 patients 12–50 months after the rupture of an ACoA aneurysm no single patient with a postoperative Korsakoff syndrome. Two patients were, however, aphasic. In 3–15 (9–47%) patients cognitive deficits were found. Memory deficits in the Rey-Osterrieth task were most prominent with 47% (Teissier du Cros and Lhermitte, 1984). Alexander and Freedman (1984) investigated 11 patients with amnesia and personality changes after rupture and surgical repair of an aneurysm of the

ACoA neuropsychologically. All patients demonstrated postoperative disturbances of initiative, confabulations and anosognosia. In four patients the confabulations persisted in the long run. Except for two patients, all exhibited infarcts. One of the patients without infarction had a left-frontal arteriovenous malformation (AVM). In two patients the infarcts were localized parietally, the others exhibited frontal infarctions (Alexander and Freedman, 1984). In the light of these results, it becomes evident that patients with amnesias and confabulations after the rupture and operative therapy of an ACoA aneurysm generally also exhibited frontal and/or parietal infarcts.

In a small group study, Corkin et al. (1985) investigated patients with global amnesia after the rupture of an ACoA aneurysm and compared these to 13 amnestics of other etiology (closed head injury, Korsakoff psychosis, stroke, herpes simplex encephalitis, anoxia and bilateral temporal lobe resection). The authors pointed out the restricted comparability of the different etiological groups but entertained the hypothesis that all patients presented with overlapping brain lesions (Corkin et al., 1985). The respective anatomical or morphological proofs (CCT; MRI) are, however, missing. The patients were investigated by means of an extraordinarily extensive neuropsychological test battery. Exclusively the ACoA patients showed no impairment of general intelligence and reached significantly higher IQ values than all other patients. Furthermore, in comparison to the other groups, the ACoA patients exhibited the smallest frequency of cognitive deficits. In a single case study, Parkin, Leng and Stanhope (1988) investigated a patient after rupture and surgery on an ACoA aneurysm using a variety of neuropsychological tests with special emphasis on memory functions. Surgery proved to be difficult and a CCT scan performed nine months later showed an enlarged left anterior horn with a hypointensity adjacent to the lateral ventricle. Postoperatively, a psychoorganic syndrome lasting for more than one year, consisting of amnesia, disorientation and completely lacking insight into the own impairments (anosognosia), occurred. Neuropsychological investigation, carried out two years later revealed an above average general IQ but a substantially worse performance in the WMS. No deficits in the WCST and in a word fluency task were found. The results of the numerous memory tasks were interpreted such by the authors that ACoA patients with amnesia are especially susceptible to interference (Parkin, Leng and Stanhope, 1988). DeLuca (1992b) reported about two cases who developed a Korsakoff syndrome with amnesia and confabulation after rupture and surgical treatment of an ACoA aneurysm. Furthermore, disturbances of executive functions and slight to moderate personality changes were observed (DeLuca, 1992b).

10.3.3. The significance of frontal brain damage for amnestic syndromes after rupture and surgery for an ACoA aneurysm

Steinman and Bigler (1986) investigated a small group of 7 patients after the rupture of an ACoA aneurysm by means of an extensive neuropsychological test battery. Furthermore, changes of personality and behavioral disturbances were recorded. Exceptionally, all patients had a bilateral frontomesial infarction which encompassed in two of them both anterior parts of both hemispheres as the consequence of massive intracerebral hemorrhage (Steinman and Bigler, 1986). Despite the considerable morphological damage, in all patients general intelligence was unimpaired. Furthermore, no perceptive disturbances, visual field defects or apraxias were found. On the other hand, all patients except for one had substantial deficits in the WMS. One further patient presented with global aphasia. The most frequent neuropsychological impairment was in five of six patients an impairment in the Category Test for abstraction capacity and cognitive flexibility. Behavioral disturbances and emotional disorders were seen, however, in 54–100% of the patients (Steinman and Bigler, 1986). The authors concluded from their results that after the rupture of an ACoA aneurysm general intellectual capacities are left relatively intact while deficits of short-term memory and personality changes ensue. This conclusion was explained such that due to the rupture of an ACoA aneurysm especially fronto-limbic hypothalamic circuits of the basal forebrain are disturbed. The frequent personality disturbances could then be regarded as an expression of frontal brain damage (Steinman and Bigler, 1986). Apart from the unusual morphological damage of the study sample of Steinman and Bigler (1986), most of all the postulated association to the rupture of an ACoA aneurysm cannot be kept up, since also patients with ruptured aneurysms of other locations exhibit a similar pattern of neuropsychological impairments (Hütter and Gilsbach, 1996a; 1992; Hütter, Gilsbach and Kreitschmann, 1995; Satzger et al., 1995; Tidswell et al., 1995; Ogden et al., 1993a; DeLuca, 1993; 1992a;b; Richardson, 1991; 1989).

In a single case study, Leng and Parkin (1988) compared patients with amnesia after ACoA aneurysm rupture and a fronto-orbital infarction with seven Korsakoff patients and five patients who had developed amnesia after herpes simplex encephalitis, with respect to their performance in a number of tests, generally regarded as sensitive for frontal brain function. Also the patients after the rupture of an ACoA aneurysm showed abnormalities, which were interpreted by the authors as an indicator for fronto-cortical cognitive dysfunction (Leng and Parkin, 1988). In contrast, the patterns of the fronto-cortical cognitive dysfunctions differed between the etiological groups (Leng and Parkin, 1988).

Shoqeirat et al. (1990) compared five patients with amnesia after the rupture of an ACoA aneurysm with 10 amnestics after herpes simplex encephalitis and 16 patients with an alcohol induced Korsakoff syndrome. The patients after encephalitis performed significantly better in the WCST than the other patients (Shoqeirat et al., 1990). Although difficult to comprehend in view of the presented data, the authors concluded from their results that in amnestics, regardless of etiology, indications for frontal brain damage are present (Shoqeirat et al., 1990). It is difficult to draw a clear conclusion from the interpretation of the data of Shoqeirat et al. (1990), since the study sample consisted of a group of 31 randomly collected amnestics, and it is in no case mandatory that frontal brain damage constitutes a necessary prerequisite for the occurrence of an amnestic disturbance. In a further study, Shoqeirat and Mayes (1991) investigated the memory function of 17 amnestics with alcohol induced Korsakoff syndrome, after a herpes simplex encephalitis or after the rupture of and surgery for an ACoA aneurysm with special regard to spatial memory. All patients in the three etiological groups presented with comparable impairments of spatial memory performance. The deficits of spatial memory showed no association at all to fronto-cortical dysfunctions, while the considerable deficits in free recall, which could be found in all groups, showed no correlation to spatial memory, but were substantially dependent on the age of the patients and on the degree of impairment of frontal brain function (Shoqeirat and Mayes, 1991). These results demonstrate, that spatial memory and recall processes constitute two different relatively independent memory systems and processes of free recall seem to be connected to frontal brain function.

DeLuca and Cicerone (1991) compared the frequency and pattern of confabulations in nine ACoA patients to those of 17 patients with spontaneous intracranial bleedings of different etiology. CCT results were available in eight ACoA patients, four of whom had infarcts visible on CCT. In two further patients neuroradiological signs of acute hydrocephalus were present. A further two patients presented with frontal hygromas. The ACoA patients were investigated neuropsychologically in the subacute stage of their illness between three and 16 weeks after the acute event. Confabulatory amnesia was present in all patients of the ACoA group while only seven of the 17 patients in the other group showed confabulations. The authors concluded from these findings that in ACoA patients, the involvement of the frontal lobe promotes the occurrence of confabulations (DeLuca and Cicerone, 1991).

On the contrary, the results of DeLuca (1990) who described a patient presenting with frontal infarcts but was neither amnestic nor presented with confabulations point in a different direction. In order to resolve this contradiction, DeLuca (1993) proposed that damage to two separate areas, namely the basal forebrain and frontal lobe damage must coincide in order to induce confabulations. This hypothesis is supported, at least in part, by the results of Irle et al. (1992a), who found that patients with lesions of the basal forebrain and the striatum presented with substantial memory deficits while the amnestic disturbances of patients with different lesions or combinations of lesions, respectively, were not as severe. In a further single case study, DeLuca (1993) compared three patients with amnesia after the rupture of an ACoA aneurysm to three further patients without amnesia after the rupture of an ACoA aneurysm. All six patients exhibited frontal abnormalities on CCT with two of the three non-amnestic patients presenting with frontal intracerebral hemorrhage. In none of the non-amnestic patients, confabulations occurred. These results illustrate that neither the rupture of an ACoA aneurysm nor frontal brain damage are necessary nor sufficient prerequisites for the occurrence of amnesias and/or confabulations. DeLuca (1993) hence concluded that possibly frontal brain damage together with an amnestic syndrome form the prerequisite for confabulations. The results of DeLuca (1993) also demonstrate, however, that after rupture and surgical repair of an ACoA aneurysm such cognitive and behavioral abnormalities that correspond to an ACoA syndrome must not necessarily occur. In so far, no causal relationship between these abnormalities and ACoA aneurysm location exists.

Vilkki (1985) investigated five patients with amnesias after rupture and surgical repair of an ACoA aneurysm. Although two patients presented with amnesia, postoperative CCT showed no frontal abnormalities. Therefore, Vilkki (1985) concluded that after rupture and surgery for an ACoA aneurysm amnesia can occur without frontal brain damage. On the other hand, a confusional state or Korsakoff-like confabulations require manifest frontal brain damage next to an amnestic syndrome (Vilkki, 1985). Already Stuss et al. (1978) postulated that the confabulations of ACoA patients result of an impairment of frontal brain functions which is accompanied by a considerable memory disturbance. In a retrospective study, Thomas-Anterion et al. (1995) compared seven patients with an amnestic syndrome which had become manifest after surgery for an ACoA aneurysm to 11 patients without an amnestic syndrome after surgical repair of an ACoA aneurysm as well as 18 controls with respect to their performance in a neuropsychological test battery. Most patients had been operated upon late (>72 hours) and only few were in a clinical state worse than grade II according to Hunt and Hess on admission to the hospital (Thomas-Anterion et al., 1995). In the amnestics, evidence for frontal dysfunction in the Stroop Test which did not differ in severity from the non-amnestic ACoA patients and a deficit in the retrieval process were revealed. On the other hand, in no patient a manifest frontal lobe syndrome was present. In both patient groups, procedural memory was undisturbed. Some amnestics additionally presented with anosognosia for their deficits. The authors concluded from their results that in patients after rupture and surgical repair of an ACoA aneurysm fronto-cortical cognitive impairment of function oftentimes occurs independent of the presence of an amnestic syndrome and does not become manifest as a frontal lobe syndrome. Rather, according to the opinion of Thomas-Anterion et al. (1995), fronto-cortical functional impairment remains largely subliminal.

Van der Linden et al. (1993) investigated eight amnestic ACoA patients 4–48 months after surgery and a control group with respect to the susceptibility for proactive interference (PI). Additionally, the patients were investigated by means of a short version of the WCST, a Stroop Test and a word fluency task. The ACoA patients exhibited a significantly larger susceptibility for PI and performed significantly worse in all tests of frontal brain function (WCST, Stroop Test and word fluency task) than the controls (Van der Linden et al., 1993). Moreover, a significant correlation between the Stroop Test and errors in the PI task emerged, pointing to a connection between frontal brain functions and the susceptibility for interference in memory tasks. However, the results are not surprising, since in the study of Van der Linden et al. (1993), all ACoA patients presented with frontal brain damage on CCT which often coincides with impaired frontal brain function. When interpreting these results, it must be considered that frontal brain damage visible on CCT is only observed in 9% of all ACoA patients. Therefore, the study sample of Van der Linden et al. (1993) contains an unusual accumulation of patients with frontal brain damage, so that no generalized conclusions pertaining to the entire collective of ACoA patients can be drawn. As these examples show, psychorganic impairments after rupture and surgical treatment of an ACoA aneurysm can often be the result of damage to diencephalic and/or frontal structures caused by the hemorrhage itself, vasospasm or the surgical intervention. From a functional-neuropsychological point of view, Volpe and Hirst (1983) postulated, that the memory disturbances of patients with ruptured ACoA aneurysms are often caused by increased susceptibility to interference, which again would speak in favor of fronto-cortical dysfunction. In two older studies on the sequelae of the rupture and operative treatment of ACoA aneurysms, next to confabulatory memory disturbance, the patients presented with additional deficits in those neuropsychological tests supposed to measure frontal brain function even though they did not exhibit visible morphological frontal brain damage (Alexander and Freedman, 1984; Kapur and Coughlan, 1980). The authors concluded thereof that the frontal lesions did not necessarily have to be so extensive as to be visible on CCT scans (Alexander and Freedman, 1984; Kapur and Coughlan, 1980).

10.3.4. The neuroanatomical basis of the neuropsychological abnormalities after rupture and surgical repair of aneurysms of the ACoA

In two patients with chronic amnesia after the rupture of an ACoA aneurysm three years after the ictus, Volpe, Herscovitch and Raichle (1984) found a hypometabolism in both mesial temporal lobes but not in fronto-orbital or thalamic areas using O_2-PET. This finding supports the hypothesis that the anatomical distribution of blood in the basal cisterns plays an important role in the etiology of the neuropsychological impairments after SAH (also see Table 1, Chapter 4). Damasio et al. (1985a) reviewed the cases of six patients with ACoA aneurysms and localized damage in the orbito-frontal and basal forebrain using surgical reports, intraoperative photographs as well as imaging diagnostics such as CCT and SPECT. In the patients, damage to the gyrus rectus, the septal nuclei, the nucleus accumbens, the substantia innominata and associated fiber tracts as the precommissural fornix were found (Damasio et al., 1985a). The amnestic syndromes encompassed before all the retrieval process and were accompanied by considerable changes of personality. The authors concluded from the data, that damage to the basal forebrain leads to a decoupling of the hippocampus and, therefore, interrupts or minimizes the cholinergic innervation of large cortical areas (Damasio et al., 1985a).

A very interesting and informative case report on the neuropsychological sequelae of the rupture and surgical repair of an ACoA aneurysm in a 37-year old patient stems from Philips, Sangalang and Sterns (1987). Due to the death of the patient, it had become possible to perform a neuropathological investigation five years after an extensive neurological, neuroradiological and neuropsychological investigation. Angiography revealed next to the aneurysm that the proximal portion of the right ACA did not contrast. Fourteen days later the aneurysm was clipped and wrapped after right frontal craniotomy. Immediately postoperatively, the patient presented with a severe confusional state combined with anterograde amnesia and lack of initiative which persisted until his death five years later. Postoperatively, a diabetes insipidus as well as disturbances of the sodium metabolism with intermittent hypo- and hyper-natremia as an indicator for hypothalamic damage developed. Neuropsychological investigation revealed inconspicuous test results in nearly all areas as well as a normal IQ. Only in the memory tasks considerable impairments were found. Working memory seemed intact, but already after a short span of time, recall of material learnt shortly before was not possible. A repeated neuropsychological assessment after 28 months revealed for the most part unchanged results, however, new extensive deficits became evident in working memory and the WCST. This secondary worsening of performance might be explained first by the occurrence of hydrocephalus and second by secondary tissue degeneration as a consequence of the primary brain damage (Hütter, Mayfrank and Gilsbach, submitted).

Neuropathological investigation demonstrated hemosiderin impregnation of the right gyrus rectus, the paraolfactory hypothalamic areas and the suprasellar cistern which substantiates damage to this area by the bleeding itself. These findings do not explain, however, the neuropsychological impairments of the patient, since these became evident immediately postoperatively. A cystic necrotic area was found at the neuropathological investigation in the precommissural grey, the diagonal band of Broca, the nucleus accumbens, a small rostro-ventral portion of the globus pallidus and a ventral segment of the anterior part of the internal capsule. The anterior commissure, the postcommissural grey and the nucleus basalis Meynert were, however, left intact (Philips, Sangalang and Sterns, 1987). Consequently, the bleeding itself, surgery or secondary complications such as vasospasm may account for the above described morphological damage. Since the affected structures exhibit far-reaching connections to limbic areas, temporal and thalamic structures, the abnormalities observed in the patient, as lack of initiative in combination with memory deficits, are explainable. Yet, other already discussed causes cannot be excluded in the complex pathophysiological chain of events in the wake of an SAH. Thus, in animal experimental studies as well as in some case reports in humans, especially the nucleus of the diagonal band of Broca, the nuclei at the origin of the striae terminalis, the nuclei of the septum and the medial forebrain bundle (MFB) have been linked to functions of initiative and memory (Morecraft, Geula and Mesulam, 1993;

Mesulam, 1990; 1985; Damasio, Tranel and Damasio, 1989; Damasio et al., 1985b; Markowitsch, 1984; Wallesch et al., 1983).

DeLuca (1992b) compared the neuropsychological test performance of 11 patients after rupture of an ACoA aneurysm with that of 13 patients, who had sustained intracranial hemorrhage of other etiology. Surprisingly, in most memory tests, no difference between the two groups was found. The ACoA patients only performed significantly worse in delayed verbal recall and the WCST (DeLuca, 1992b). The author interpreted his results to the effect that ACoA aneurysm rupture does not lead to diffuse but to specific brain damage, affecting before all anterior cerebral structures. However, it is not so as postulated by DeLuca (1992b), that frontally enhanced brain damage after SAH is the specific consequence of the rupture of ACoA aneurysms but can also be the result of the rupture of aneurysms of other locations. Possibly, this also holds true for a spontaneous non-traumatic SAH without a proven source of the bleeding (Hütter, Gilsbach and Kreitschmann, 1994).

DeLuca (1992b) illustrated his conclusions with the observation that in his study patients with ruptured aneurysms of the ACoA performed significantly worse in the WCST which is sensitive for frontal brain functions. However, the patients in the ACoA group in the study of DeLuca (1992b) exhibited frontal abnormalities as seen on CCT in 6 of 10 cases (60%). In a consecutive series of aneurysm patients, in 23% infarcts or hypodensities were found on CCT, whereas only in 9% of the patients abnormalities in frontal areas were detected (Hornyak, Harders and Gilsbach, 1991). Already in an older study, Weisberg (1985) found in his patients with ruptured ACoA aneurysms three days after the bleeding in only 14% frontal infarcts on CCT. According to the data of Weisberg (1985), 22% of the ruptured ACoA aneurysms bled into the cavum septi pellucidi and 15% into the anterior interhemispheric fissure, yet also ICA or MCA aneurysms may lead to a similar bleeding pattern. In general, the rupture of an ACoA aneurysm causes, however, a symmetric hemorrhage into the basal cisterns (Weisberg, 1985). In so far, the results of DeLuca (1992b) are based on an atypical group of ACoA patients. Moreover, two patients in the sample of DeLuca (1992b) showed signs of an apparently untreated acute hydrocephalus. Therefore, it is not surprising that the patients in the study of DeLuca (1992b) performed significantly worse in the WCST. Furthermore, the control sample of DeLuca (1992b) consisted of eight patients with very unusual aneurysm locations, patients with spontaneous intracerebellar hemorrhage and of patients with hemorrhage of ruptured AV-malformations, which are not comparable to aneurysm ruptures.

Irle et al. (1992a) compared 30 patients after the rupture of mostly ACoA aneurysms with a normal CCT to 37 patients with ruptured ACoA aneurysms and abnormalities on CCT as well as to a control group. The patients with abnormalities on CCT performed significantly worse in a number of neuropsychological tests than those exhibiting normal CCT scans. In contrast to the interpretation of the authors, no indicators for a specific ACoA syndrome can be found in the results of Irle et al. (1992a). The patients with lesions in the basal forebrain or the striatum did not exhibit more but rather significantly less cognitive deficits including functions of memory in comparison to patients with lesions in the basal forebrain and the striatum and/or the ventral frontal cortex (Irle et al., 1992a). This result is difficult to interpret taking into account a number of studies and neuroanatomic-functional considerations according to which already singular lesions in the basal forebrain may lead to substantial memory disturbances and emotional changes (Damasio et al., 1985a; Damasio, Tranel and Damasio, 1989; Markowitsch, 1984; Wallesch et al., 1983). On the other hand, the findings of Irle et al. (1992a) are also difficult to interpret simply because of the fact that the morphological damage after SAH is indeed much more complex than assumed because it may encompass lesions beyond those visible on CCT. Moreover, the method of CCT analysis used by Irle et al. (1992a) has not been verified in terms of accuracy. Here, the particular problem exists that after surgical repair of an ACoA aneurysm, especially fronto-basal damage is not visible or cannot be localized reliably, respectively, because of the clip artefacts. Also, data on the comparability of the groups with respect to clinical, neuroradiological and sociodemographic variables are missing. This is a further weakness of the findings of Irle et al. (1992a). In several other studies no clear neuropsychological effects of lesions visible on CCT or MRI in patients after SAH could be demonstrated (Vilkki et al., 1990;1989; Romner et al., 1989).

Neuroanatomical studies have demonstrated a blood supply of structures in the vicinity of the anterior wall of the third ventricle by perforators emanating from the ACoA (Gomez et al., 1986; Crowell and Morawetz, 1977; Perlmutter and Rhoton, 1976). These perforators, oftentimes originating medially from the ACoA in the anterior direction, supply the anterior hypothalamus, the septum pellucidum, anterior parts of the gyrus cinguli, parts of the fornix and anterior parts of the corpus callosum including the anterior commissure (Vincentelli et al., 1991; Marinkovic, Milisavljevic and Marinkovic, 1990). Investigations by Hussein and Archilli (1996) resulted in a further anatomical specification of the main area of supply of the perforators originating from the ACoA. Hussein and Archilli (1996) were able to show that the perforators originating from the ACoA predominantly supply the nucleus basalis Meynert. Next to its function as a motor relay station, a critical importance for memory processes and the development of a brain organic psychosyndrome is ascribed to this structure (Richardson and DeLong, 1988; Damasio et al., 1985a;b). After lesions of the basal nucleus of Meynert, amnestic syndromes up to global amnesia have been described on a regular basis (Mesulam, 1990; Richardson and DeLong, 1988; Damasio et al., 1985a;b). Also further cognitive deficits beyond memory functions have been reported (Guillard, Fenelon and Mahieux, 1991).

These results enlighten the neuroanatomical basis for the postoperative amnestic syndromes, described in earlier studies in ACoA patients.

Therefore, it can be postulated that the introduction of the operating microscope and modern aneurysm clips has allowed neurosurgeons to spare the small perforators originating from the ACoA. In succession, the risk of the patient to sustain a postoperative memory deficit up to a Korsakoff syndrome has greatly diminished (Hütter and Gilsbach, 1996a; 1992; Gade, 1982). Direct empirical evidence for the significance of different surgical techniques in aneurysm surgery for the neuropsychological impairments of patients with ruptured ACoA aneurysm has first been published by Gade (Gade, 1982). The author found a close relationship between the intraoperative use of the trapping procedure of the ACoA and postoperative memory disturbances. When the aneurysm had been excluded by trapping the parent vessel, 9 (81%) of 11 patients exhibited a postoperative amnestic syndrome. Of the 37 patients in whom it had been possible to exclude the neck of the ACoA aneurysm from circulation by ligature, only in 6 (16%) cases postoperative amnesia was found (Gade, 1982).

Therefore, secondary consequences of SAH such as other kinds of surgical damage, ischemic vasospasm, subacute brain edema and, most of all, the bleeding itself with its different pathogenic aspects remain the most important causes for the cognitive and psychosocial impairments of ACoA patients. In so far, the anatomical pattern of the bleeding must be taken increasingly into account when investigating the neuropsychological sequelae of the rupture of an ACoA aneurysm in the future.

10.3.5. Group studies on the neuropsychological sequelae of the rupture and surgical repair of aneurysms of the ACoA

In a series of recent studies which at least partly fulfill the required methodological standards, neither massive impairments of memory functions nor more cognitive impairments in general could be substantiated in ACoA patients. Table 1 gives an overview of those studies in which no difference between the cognitive deficits of ACoA patients and patients after the rupture of aneurysms of other locations could be found.

In a study by Vilkki et al. (1989), patients after rupture and surgical repair of an ACoA aneurysm did not perform worse than patients after rupture of an intracranial aneurysm of other locations. Only one patient showed a persisting postoperative amnesia together with a Korsakoff syndrome (Vilkki et al., 1989). Richardson (1989) could not find a statistically significant difference in the postoperative impairment in a number of tasks for the assessment of verbal recall between patients with ruptured aneurysms of different locations including the ACoA. However, Richardson (1989) did not analyze his data especially in respect of the effect of ACoA aneurysm location and did not formulate a specific hypothesis related to this patient group. Moreover, Richardson (1989) only tested a relatively small and specific aspect of different memory functions with the assessment of verbal recall. Since no effect of aneurysm localization on the performance in word fluency tasks could be substantiated, a preferential

Table 1. Studies in which no differences in the neuropsychological test performance between ACoA patients and patients with ruptured aneurysms at other locations were found

Author(s)	Journal	Year of publication
Richardson	Brain and Cognition	1989
Vilkki et al.	Neurosurgery	1989
Hütter & Gilsbach	Acta Neurochir (Wien)	1992
DeLuca	J Clin Exp Neuropsychol	1992
Ogden et al.	Neurosurgery	1993
Hütter & Gilsbach	J Clin Exp Neuropsychol	1995
Satzger et al.	Acta Neurochir (Wien)	1995
Tidswell et al.	Neurology	1995
Hütter & Gilsbach	Acta Neurochir (Wien)	1996
Hütter[1]	Neuropsychiatry Neuropsychol Behav Neurol	1998

[1]In this study only the psychologic adjustment had been explored

damage to frontal structures due to the rupture of an ACoA aneurysm is unlikely and just as well possible as a consequence of the rupture of aneurysms of other locations (Richardson, 1989).

Laiacona et al. (1989) investigated 43 patients 7–101 months after rupture and surgical repair of an ACoA aneurysm with respect to their cognitive deficits. In all patients the right gyrus rectus had been resected. Furthermore, hypotension had been initiated intraoperatively when deemed necessary and all patients were treated antifibrinolytically. It is meanwhile known of such measures that they constitute risk factors for additional damage to the patient (Kreitschmann-Andermahr and Gilsbach, 1996). In 68% of the patients abnormalities were seen on CCT and 35% exhibited substantial persisting cognitive impairments with impairments of verbal short-term memory found in 23% as the most frequent deficit. Laiacona et al. (1989) stressed that amnestic disturbances were found far less often in their study sample than would have been expected according to the scientific literature. Moreover, deficits of short-term memory occurred more frequently than impairments of longer term memory functions. The authors concluded from their results that the pattern of found deficits did not exhibit anything typical for the ACoA localization and that, instead, oftentimes cognitive deficits emerged which had not been expected in connection with this aneurysm location (Laiacona et al., 1989). Hampl et al. (1990) investigated 135 patients 1–7 years after aneurysm rupture by means of a neuropsychological test battery. No significant difference was found between the 47% of the patients with a ruptured ACoA aneurysm and the patients with other aneurysm locations (Hampl et al., 1990). Gade and Mortensen (1990) compared 20 amnestics after surgery for an ACoA aneurysm with 19 amnestics of mixed etiology (tumor, hemorrhage, encephalitis, Korsakoff syndrome, anoxia etc.) and 19 patients with dementias of different etiology with respect to the frequency and severity of retrograde amnesias. No difference between the etiological groups pertaining to the retrograde amnesias could be demonstrated.

Stenhouse et al. (1991) investigated 27 patients 12–84 months after surgery for a ruptured ACoA aneurysm in order to identify persisting neuropsychological abnormalities. All patients had been operated upon late. The Wechsler Intelligence Test, the WMS and the WCST were used. Among the 59% patients with cognitive deficits, six (22%) were identified with a severe general cognitive impairment and a further 8 (30%) exhibited deficits, most of all in the WCST which points to a marked impairment of fronto-cortical cognitive functions (Stenhouse et al., 1991). Maurice-Williams et al. (1991) also did not find any relationship between postoperative impairments of cognitive performance capacity and the ACoA aneurysm location, without performing, however, a concise group comparison.

In the study by Hütter and Gilsbach (1992) the neuropsychological test performance of 18 patients after rupture and early surgery for an ACoA aneurysm was compared to that of 21 patients with ruptured aneurysms of other locations and 9 patients after spontaneous non-traumatic SAH of unknown origin. Both groups were comparable with respect to age, distance in time to the acute event, neurological state on admission to the hospital (Hunt and Hess) and the severity of the SAH (Fischer CCT grading). Nevertheless, a statistically insignificant tendency toward more frequent intracerebral and/or intraventricular hemorrhages in the ACoA patient group was identified. The neurological result at the time of six-month follow-up corresponded to GOS = I or GOS = II. The ACoA patients neither differed significantly from the control group in terms of the frequency of cognitive impairments nor in the mean scores of all neuropsychological tests (Hütter and Gilsbach, 1992). In the study by Hütter and Gilsbach (1992) one to five years after the acute event, in no single one of the 18 patients in the ACoA group, global amnesia and/or Korsakoff-like confabulations, as observed frequently in earlier studies, was present (Volpe and Hirst, 1983; Okawa et al., 1980; Nyström, 1973; Talland, Sweet and Ballantine, 1967; Lindquist and Norlen, 1966; Talland, 1960). Even in the acute stage of the illness, few days (median 5 days) after early surgery no substantial differences between the mean test scores of 13 patients after rupture of an ACoA aneurysm and 15 patients after clipping of aneurysms of other locations were found (Hütter and Gilsbach, 1996a). Table 2 shows the comparison of the mean test scores between the two patient groups.

In a study on the quality of life and cognitive deficits of patients in the chronic state after SAH, no statistically significant differences in the frequency of self- and proxy-rated impairments in daily life between patients with ruptured ACoA aneurysms and patients with ruptured intracranial aneurysms of other locations or a spontaneous non-traumatic SAH without a proven source of the bleeding emerged (Hütter, Gilsbach and Kreitschmann, 1995). Moreover, in a further study, no relationship between ACoA aneurysm location and impaired capacity for introspection was found

Table 2. Neuropsychological test performance of the ACoA patients and of the patients with ruptured aneurysms at other locations

	ACoA group		Other aneurysm location/no aneurysm			
	n = 13		n = 15		t-test	
Tests	mean	SD	mean	SD	F	p
Token Test[1]	3,4	5,4	3,2	5,1	1,12	0,92 ns
d2 speed[2]	95,2	13,4	99,6	7,8	2,93	0,32 ns
d2 error %[2]	4,2	2,4	4,3	2,8	1,37	0,90 ns
d2 error-reduced[2]	93,4	14,4	97,2	8,7	2,73	0,42 ns
IST-Memory[3]	89,6	7,5	91,6	7,6	1,03	0,49 ns
Benton test[4]	5,2	2,3	4,8	2,1	1,22	0,66 ns
Reaction-time[5]	294,7	107,7	304,1	122,2	1,29	0,86 ns
Alertness[5]	54,0	9,6	52,1	14,9	2,39	0,76 ns
Div. attention[5] (reaction-time)	747,1	104,3	704,2	138,3	1,76	0,49 ns
Div. attention[5] (omissions)	4,2	4,4	4,0	4,0	1,16	0,90 ns

ns = not significant
[1]Aphasia screening test: No. of errors; [2]Test of concentration d2: standard values/stanine values; [3]Long-term memory: standard values; [4]Short-term memory: no. of correct reproductions; [5]Zimmermann testing battery: reaction times in milliseconds (msec) age-adjusted raw scores; Alertness: T-values, Div. = divided attention: No. of omissions, raw scores according to Hütter and Gilsbach (1996a)

(Hütter and Gilsbach, 1995a). Also Satzger et al. (1995) found no difference in the neuropsychological test performance between patients with ruptured ACoA aneurysms and patients with ruptured aneurysms of other locations. In a study by Ogden, Utley and Mee (1997) in a sample of 123 patients four to seven years after SAH, no difference emerged between patients after rupture of an ACoA aneurysm and the other patients in self-rated memory performance capacity. In a further study on psychological adjustment of patients after rupture and early surgery of an ACoA aneurysm, the patients in the ACoA group presented with a comparable degree of psychological problems as patients with spontaneous SAH of other etiology (Hütter, 1998). This result is distinguished from earlier studies in which ACoA patients showed particularly distinct emotional disturbances (Alexander and Freedman, 1984; Kapur and Coughlan, 1980; Okawa et al., 1980; Sengupta, Chinu and Brierley, 1975).

In sum, these negative results can be interpreted as a sequel of the improved modern neurosurgical management of subarachnoid hemorrhage due to aneurysm rupture, such as the introduction of the operating microscope, modern aneurysm clips, the discontinuance of the trapping procedure of the aneurysm bearing vessel, the introduction of the calcium antagonist nimodipine, transcranial Doppler sonography (TCD), a specialized intensive care and pharmacological management and the principle of early surgery (Hütter et al., 1999; Gilsbach et al., 1990; Gilsbach and Harders, 1989; Gilsbach et al., 1988a).

11. Impairments in daily life after SAH

Contemporary social medicine differentiates three levels of effects of bodily illnesses: 1. "impairment" as the injured organ system, 2. "disability" as the resulting impaired function and 3. "handicap" as the individual psychosocial consequences (World Health Organization, 1980). Next to the level of neuropsychological impairments which should correspond to disability, the psychosocial impairments are to be mentioned on the handicap level. Although an illness such as SAH often leads to permanent disturbances of brain function, visible bodily impairments are rare. Therefore, it could be termed a "hidden" illness. The consequences of the illness cannot be observed directly by outsiders since no visible impairments or other abnormalities show in the outer appearance of the patient. Six months after the acute event only 20% of all patients exhibit deficits noticeable for outsiders such as pareses or mental impairments as severe aphasias (Gilsbach and Harders, 1989). Nevertheless, the patients are substantially handicapped in their daily functional capacity. Therefore, also in patients after SAH also questions about problems in daily life are of great importance. Based on the brain organic limitation to perceive the own deficits and because of the fact that assessments by the life-companion are in general more reliable, also the patients' partners should be questioned about complaints and functional impairments (Hütter and Gilsbach, 1995a). For this reason it is sensible, also in scientific studies, to take the assessment of the state of the patient by the life-companion (proxy-rating) into account (Hütter and Gilsbach, 1996b; 1995a;b; Hütter, Gilsbach and Kreitschmann, 1995).

Artiola, Fortuny and Prieto-Valiente (1981) investigated 204 patients after aneurysm rupture by means of a follow-up questionnaire. The authors determined that the frequency of physical dependency and psychiatric abnormalities exhibited no correlation with the location of the aneurysm when the effect of other clinical variables was controlled for (Artiola, Fortuny and Prieto-Valiente, 1981). McKenna et al. (1989a) found a considerable number of patients after SAH with substantial impairments in daily life. Thus, 80% of the patients exhibited an impairment in at least one area of function (McKenna et al., 1989a). However, the authors reduced this rate arbitrarily by integrating a proxy-rating designed to eliminate such complaints which could not be attributed immediately to the illness. This procedure is difficult to follow in two respects, since for once the validity of the correction process is per se questionable and, second, a critical life event causes further events which result not directly but indirectly of the primary critical life event (Kessler, Price and Wortman, 1985). As a salient result of their study, McKenna et al. (1989a) pointed out that one year after the hemorrhage patients complained of increased tiredness. The patients' greatest fear was to sustain a second hemorrhage. Furthermore, headache proved to be a frequent problem and stressed the patients severely. However, data on the frequency and severity of these impairments are unfortunately not given by McKenna et al. (1989a).

Vilkki et al. (1990) investigated 83 patients one year after their aneurysm rupture by means of neuropsychological tests and an interview pertaining to complaints in everyday life. Additionally, a CCT scan was performed in every patient. No differences in the cognitive status were found between emotionally impaired and the unimpaired patients. Also the social adjustment of the patients could not be predicted reliably on the basis of their neuropsychological test performance. In patients with left-sided infarcts and/or diffuse brain damage, reintegration into employment was worse, while patients with right-sided infarcts complained of more cognitive impairments and, furthermore, exhibited more anxiety and depression (Vilkki et al., 1990). Hütter, Gilsbach and Kreitschmann (1995) found that approximately 50% of the patients one to five years after SAH reported of a significant deterioration in different areas of their daily life. This opinion was mostly shared by the patients' life companions. In the study of Hütter, Gilsbach and Kreitschmann (1995), according to the patients' self-rating, quality of life after the SAH had worsened significantly before all in the areas of concentration capacity (70%), free-time activities (52%), motivation (50%), interest in events of daily life (47%), mental capacity (47%), sleep (47%), social contact (39%) and, to a lesser extent, in the area of motor fine coordination (25%). No significant differences in the mean scores of the individual ratings between patients and partners, between operated patients and those with SAH without proven source of the bleeding and between patients with a ruptured ACoA aneurysm versus those with ruptured aneurysms of other locations could be established (Hütter, Gilsbach and Kreitschmann, 1995). Comparable subjective complaints were also found in other studies where patients complained of increased fatigue, distractibility and irritability (Ogden, Uttley and Mee, 1997; Tidswell et al., 1995; Ogden, Mee and Henning, 1993a; Vilkki et al., 1990; Sonesson et al., 1989; 1987; Bornstein et al., 1987; Ljunggren et al., 1985). Ljunggren et al. (1985) found that deficits in memory functions and lack of cognitive flexibility in SAH patients were typically associated with the inability to regain full working capacity and impaired social contacts even if the neurological recovery was complete. Vilkki et al. (1990; 1989) reported similar results in a sample of 83 patients after SAH.

Ogden, Mee and Henning (1994) investigated 66 patients one year after SAH by means of a clinical interview and a series of questionnaires. The most frequent impairments reported were considerably increased tiredness by 86% of the patients and oversensitivity against loud noise by 55% of the patients. In 8–19% of the patients emotional changes and in 16%

impairments in social life were noted (Ogden, Mee and Henning, 1994). The authors did not find any statistically significant differences between operated patients and those after non-traumatic SAH without a proven source of the bleeding (Ogden, Mee and Henning, 1994). Ogden, Utley and Mee (1997) investigated 121 patients between four and seven years after the acute event by means of a telephone interview or a questionnaire with respect to psychosocial changes after SAH. In 16.5–48.3% of their patients the authors found persisting subjective complaints. More than 75% of the patients reported of having suffered of considerably increased tiredness for a prolonged time after the hemorrhage which had abated within the course of some years (Ogden, Utley and Mee, 1997). Table 1 shows the frequency of impairments in daily life as reported in various studies by patients after SAH.

It must be pointed out, however, that all patients in the study of Steinman and Bigler (1986) exhibited frontal infarcts and all patients in the study of Teissier du Cros and Lhermitte (1984) had a ruptured ACoA aneurysm. Especially in the areas initiative, mental capacity, free-time activities, social contacts and emotional state, numerous patients reported unfavorable changes.

The impairments in everyday life in patients after SAH are comparable to those of patients after traumatic brain injury (Uzell, 1988; Uzell, Langfitt and Dolinskas, 1987). Already Gronwall and Wrightson (1974) discovered in their study on the neuropsychological sequelae of mild closed head injury a typical pattern of diffuse complaints consisting of tiredness, irritability, distractibility, poor concentration and headache. The authors explained this syndrome by a general decrease in information processing capacity as a consequence of the failure of the parsing process for the processing of information from several channels (Gronwall and Wrightson, 1974). This leads to the conjecture that both patient groups are impaired in functions of attention such as reaction time, speed of cognitive processing, attention capacity and selective attention. Half of the patients in the study by Hütter, Gilsbach and Kreitschmann (1995) felt physically incomplete since their SAH. Thus, their bodily self-perception had suffered permanently as a consequence of the hemorrhage. A further result of importance for improved future follow-up consists therein that 69% of the patients complained of a lack of information on their illness (Hütter, Gilsbach and Kreitschmann, 1995).

Increased headache since the time of SAH proves a frequent and stressing problem for the patient which has already been made the topic of several studies. Surprisingly, the importance of problems with headache has not been investigated further in SAH patients although it constitutes significant discomfort for the patient. Increased sensitivity to changes of weather, headache, oftentimes triggered by mental effort and agitation, were found in SAH patients in several studies (Ogden, Utley and Mee, 1997; Hütter, Gilsbach and Kreitschmann, 1995; Ruelle et al., 1985). Headache can be regarded for the one part as an expression of psychosomatic disturbance.

Table 1. Frequency of impairments in daily life following SAH

Authors	No.	Delay SAH/ Follow-up	Method	Motivation/ tiredness	Social relations	Emotional changes	Cognitive symptoms
Teissier du Cros & Lhermitte (1984)	32	11–50 months	clinical interview	34%	13%	25%	not assessed
Steinmann & Bigler (1986)	8	11 months–9 years	clinical interview	100%	66%	54%	90%
McKenna et al. (1989a)	70	1 year	clinical interview	19%	4%	33%	not assessed
Vilkki (1990)	83	1 year	clinical interview	not assessed	25%	not assessed	56%
Ogden et al. (1990)	16	5 years	clinical interview	38%	38%	not assessed	69%[1]
Stegen & Freckmann (1991)	87	1 year	proxy-rating	not assessed	23%	28%	45%
Ogden, Mee & Henning (1994)	66	1 year	clinical interview	86%	16%[3]	8–19%[3]	not assessed
Hütter et al. (1995)	58	1–5 years	questionnaire	50%	39%	36%[2]	47%
Ogden et al. (1997)	123	4–7 years	interview by phone/ questionnaire	35%	not assessed	48%	41%[4]

[1] Increased irritability
[2] Increased depression (depression inventory of Beck)
[3] Questionnaires
[4] Memory problems

On the other hand, chronic headache also constitutes a considerable psychological burden and can impair the general quality of life of the affected patients substantially. Ogden, Utley and Mee (1997) found in a sample of 123 patients 4–7 years after SAH in 17% substantial strain due to headache. Also patients after non-aneurysmal SAH are affected by increased headache. Ruelle et al. (1985) reported that 21% of the patients after non-aneurysmal SAH suffered of severe persisting headache. In the study of Hütter, Gilsbach and Kreitschmann (1995), 77% of the patients reported a considerably more frequent strain due to headache since the SAH. The significance for the emotional adjustment of the patients is emphasized by the results of Hütter, Gilsbach and Kreitschmann (1995). The frequency of headache correlated significantly with a reduced life satisfaction ($r = 0.42$; $p < 0.01$), increased bodily complaints ($r = 0.71$; $p < 0.001$) and increased emotional lability ($r = 0.46$; $p < 0.01$), as measured by the respective subscales of the FPI-R (Hütter, Gilsbach and Kreitschmann, 1995). Admittedly, a great variability of the frequency of headache within the individual studies exists which can probably explained by differences in methodology. Apart from this, headache in patients after SAH is a significant clinical and psychological problem. Therefore, a necessity for the clarification of the pathophysiological nature of this chronic stress factor after SAH as well as for the development and implementation of suitable treatment methods is given. The pathophysiological nature of this kind of headache remains unresolved, but scarring around the cerebral arteries as a consequence of the bleeding might be considered a causal factor.

12. Psychological adjustment and depression after SAH

In the chronic state after SAH, increased irritability, changes of personality, loss of interests and initiative, social problems and emotional disturbances frequently persist (Hütter, 1998; Ogden, Utley and Mee, 1997; Hütter, Gilsbach and Kreitschmann, 1995; Säveland et al., 1992; 1986; Stegen and Freckmann, 1991; Maurice-Williams et al., 1991; Vilkki et al., 1990; Sonesson et al., 1989; 1987; Bornstein et al., 1987; Ljunggren et al., 1985). These psychological disturbances and subjective complaints are also present when the degree of neurological and/or cognitive impairments is relatively mild (Hütter, 1998; Hütter, Gilsbach and Kreitschmann, 1995; Stegen and Freckmann, 1991; Vilkki et al., 1990; Ljunggren et al., 1985). Ropper and Zervas (1984) investigated a series of 112 consecutive cases after aneurysm rupture presenting with a good neurological recovery and detected in 25% of their patients substantial emotional disturbances. Ljunggren et al. (1985) reported that 25% of their SAH patients with a good neurological result (GOS = I) complained of emotional problems in a clinical interview. Säveland et al. (1986) determined that of 21 patients after SAH and aneurysm rupture 5 (24%) exhibited severe psychosocial impairments. Taking into account the neuropsychological result, in a consecutive series of 87 patients after aneurysm rupture, only 33% exhibited a good neurological and psychosocial result (Säveland et al., 1986). Bornstein et al. (1987) also found frequent emotional disturbances in SAH patients who had been investigated by means of a clinical interview and the Minnesota Multiphasic Personality Inventory (MMPI). In a further study Vilkki et al. (1990) described changes of personality and emotional problems in a sample of patients after SAH investigated by means of standardized personality tests. In 32% of the patients, Vilkki et al. (1990) found significant changes of personality. In a collective of 87 patients after SAH with a mostly good neurological recovery (GOS = I), Stegen and Freckmann (1991) observed in almost all of their patients (98%) changes in social behavior, a deteriorated mood in 51% and depression in 36% of them. Mercier et al. (1991) found in 35% of their patients three months after aneurysm rupture evidence for changes of personality and emotional disturbances. Ogden, Henning and Mee (1993a) reported that one year after SAH, mostly as a consequence of aneurysm rupture, 14.6% of their patients exhibited a clinically significant depression in the BDI. Tidswell et al. (1995) found among 37 patients after aneurysm rupture 16% with a significant depression according to the criteria of the BDI. In patients with ruptured ACoA aneurysms, a statistically insignificant trend toward a lower level of depression was seen ($p = 0.06$). Ogden, Mee and Henning (1994) found in 19% of their patients one year after the acute hemorrhage a clinically relevant depression by means of the BDI.

In a study that investigated 58 patients one to five years after SAH with respect to their problems in daily life and emotional adjustment using an adhoc questionnaire, the FPI-R and the BDI, Hütter, Gilsbach and Kreitschmann (1995) found that especially emotional lability (FPI-R) was elevated two stanine scores above the expected value in 48%. Performance motivation (FPI-R) was decreased in 41%, applying the same criterion, and life satisfaction was reduced in 37% of the patients with a value two stanine scores below the healthy normal population. No significant differences were seen between operated patients and patients with an SAH without a proven source of the bleeding. Of the 58 patients, 17 (30%) exhibited scores of > 10 in the BDI, which amounts to clinically relevant increased depressive mood. Of these, 12 (21%) exhibited a mild depression, 3 (5%) had a moderate (BDI > 20) and 2 (4%) a severe depression (BDI > 25). No differences were found between the operated and the non-operated (NA-SAH) patients and, furthermore, no effect of ACoA aneurysm location on depression emerged (Hütter, Gilsbach and Kreitschmann, 1995).

In the majority of relevant studies on psychological adjustment after SAH an adequate control group is missing by means of which could be shown in how far the abnormalities of SAH patients can be regarded as specific for the illness. Especially in the face of the persisting impairments of SAH patients, the question exists whether the often described abnormalities are a consequence of brain damage or rather an expression of chronic functional impairment. Therefore, Hütter (1998) investigated 45 patients one to five years (median 3 years) after SAH by means of a standardized questionnaire (FPI-R) with respect to their psychosocial adjustment. 36 hypoxemic patients in the end stage of chronic obstructive pulmonary disease (COPD) served as the control group. The neurological result at six-month follow-up had been assessed in 84% as good (GOS = I) and in 7 (16%) as moderate (GOS = II). In 31 (69%) patients the ruptured aneurysm had been excluded from circulation by means of early surgery (within 72 hours) while 14 (31%) patients had sustained spontaneous non-traumatic SAH without a proven source of the bleeding (Hütter, 1998). In both groups a for the most part comparable frequency of psychological disturbances was found. Only in the FPI-R subscales "bodily complaints" and "health concerns" , the COPD patients attained significantly higher scores than the SAH patients ($p < 0.05$, respectively). By means of statistical analyses, effects of gender or interactions with the variable gender could be excluded. As in earlier studies, in SAH patients loss of motivation (42%), increased introversion (40%), increased emotional lability (38%) as well as an increased feeling of strain (31%) were found especially frequently. Those patients who had been in a clinical state grade IV according to Hunt and Hess on admission to hospital showed a significantly higher loss of motivation than those patients whose clinical grade had been estimated at I–III after Hunt and Hess ($p < 0.05$). In a correlation analysis, significant correlations between the neurological state on admission to hospital (Hunt and Hess), the severity of the bleeding (Fisher CCT Score) and increased blood flow velocities (TCD) and a number of aspects of the later adjustment such as decreased social orientation (FPI-R) or increased bodily complaints (FPI-R) were found, exhibiting a size between $r = 0.32$ and $r = 0.39$ ($p < 0.01$, respectively). Table 1 gives an overview of the correlations found by Hütter (1998) between aspects of psychological adjustment (FPI-R) and a number of clinical variables in patients after SAH.

In accordance, several authors described problems of initiative as well as increased emotional lability as the most frequent psychological impairment after SAH. These, as disturbances of attention and memory can probably be explained by damage to limbic and/or frontobasal structures. They must not be visible on CCT or MRI and result of adverse effects of the subarachnoid blood on paracisternal structures.

It can be assumed that the sudden, catastrophic event SAH like "a bolt from the blue" acts as a psychological trauma that leads to the symptoms of traumatic stress disorder (American Psychiatric Association, 1994; Erikson, 1976; Horowitz, 1975). This is in line with results of the study by Stegen and Freckmann (1991), who found that 79% of their patients were afraid of recurrent hemorrhage. The aspect of psychic traumatization due to SAH offers an opportunity to explain the disparity found in this patient group

Table 1. Correlations between the FPI-R subscales and a number of clinical variables, assessed in the acute state after SAH

FPI-R subscale	Delay SAH/ Follow-up[1]	Hunt & Hess Grading	Fisher CCT-Score	Blood-flow velocities[2]
Life satisfaction	0,00 ns	−0,05 ns	−0,12 ns	0,06 ns
Social orientation	0,02 ns	0,14 ns	−0,17 ns	0,06 ns
Motivation	−0,16 ns	−0,21 ns	−0,06 ns	0,11 ns
Social insecurity	0,24 ns	0,39*	0,32*	0,36*
Ambition	−0,02 ns	−0,15 ns	−0,05 ns	0,00 ns
Aggressiveness	−0,21 ns	0,06 ns	0,08 ns	0,11 ns
Strain	−0,09 ns	−0,08 ns	−0,14 ns	−0,14 ns
Bodily disorders	−0,32*	0,17 ns	0,13 ns	0,33*
Bodily concern	0,03 ns	0,30*	0,10 ns	0,23 ns
Introversion	0,05 ns	0,06 ns	0,23 ns	0,21 ns
Emotional lability	0,01 ns	0,18 ns	0,16 ns	0,22 ns

Spearman rank order correlations
[1]Delay in years
[2]Highest mean blood-flow velocities as assessed by transcranial Doppler (TCD) independent of vessel and side (ACA, ICA, MCA) in cm/sec in the acute state after SAH
*$p < 0,05$; ns = not significant
According to Hütter (1998)

between the extent of functional impairments and the frequency of emotional disturbances. Moreover, important consequences for counseling and rehabilitation of patients after SAH would result hereof. In summary, it can be stated that the emotional disturbances after SAH are most likely the consequence of multifactorial events in which the extent of organic and cognitive impairments with their psychosocial and economic sequelae, damage to relevant brain structures, psychic traumatization, individual illness coping and an increased strain through chronic headache act together in a so far unexplained way. In this connection, the aspect of psychic traumatization represents an important new concept. These deliberations also imply that it would be desirable if illness coping and supportive measures were taken into account in future studies on the psychosocial sequelae of SAH.

13. Ability to work and professional performance capacity in patients after SAH

Next to the severity of neurological impairment, the extent of occupational reintegration and performance capacity is a further criterion often used to assess permanent sequelae of the illness and treatment success in patients after SAH. However, this criterion is subject to several limitations that impair the reliability and power of such information. Changes or regional differences of the labor market may lead to the situation that occupational reintegration of the patient is not successful although his/her functional impairments are relatively slight. Moreover, it is well known that patients with a higher level of education are more likely to return to their old profession despite considerable impairments than patients with a lower level of education. Comparable correlations should also hold true for the factors social status and professional status. Furthermore, this criterion is not applicable to housewives who still constitute a large number of the female patients, which further limits its usefulness. Lastly, the reliability of specifications on occupational reintegration remains doubtful since they are also dependent on the investigator. Additionally, it would have to be explored in detail whether eventual occupational changes or unemployment, respectively, can be attributed directly to the consequences of the illness or, if possibly other reasons are of prime importance. Only in the case of illness-dependent retirement this problem does not exist.

Logue et al. (1968) found in 79 patients (66 operated and 13 conservatively treated) after SAH that 17 (21.5%) patients could only perform light work whereas seven (8.8%) did not work because of their illness but waited for the possibility of light work and a further 11 (13.9%) patients were not able to work at all. This implies that a total of 35 (44.3%) patients in the series of Logue et al. (1968) were restricted due to their illness in their ability to work, up to the inability to work at all. Shepard et al. (1984) reported that in a sample of 254 patients with SAH without an angiographically proven aneurysm (NA-SAB), 91% of the normotensive but only 71% of the hypertensive patients reached their former working capacity. In the study of Hütter, Gilsbach and Kreitschmann (1995), in 16% of the 58 patients investigated, an illness-related occupational deterioration up to unemployment was determined on the basis of a thorough clinical interview. Since a further 15% of the patients had been retired as a consequence of the illness, 31% of the patients had sustained a substantial impairment of their professional performance capacity due to their SAH. Table 1 gives the

Table 1. Frequency of impairments of working capacity after SAH

Authors	No.	Delay SAH/ follow-up	Incapable to work	Reduced working capacity
Ruelle et al. (1985)	49	1–15 years	2%	4%
Stolke et al. (1987)	34	2–5,5 years	35%	18%
Teissier du Cros & Lhermitte (1989)	32	1 year	16%	no data
McKenna et al. (1989a)	70	1 year	24%	7%
Ogden et al. (1990)	16	5 year	no data	61%
Hampl et al. (1990)	135	1–7 years	no data	54%
Vilkki et al. (1990)	83	1 year	25%	no data
Mercier et al. (1991)	81	1–14 years	no data	31%
Ogden et al. (1993)	66	1 year	12%	26%
Hütter et al. (1995)	58	1–5 years	15%	16%
Thomas-Anterion et al. (1995)	18	1 year	no data	44%
Ogden et al. (1997)	123	4–7 years	no data	20%

Invalidity pension and unemployment as direct consequences of the illness taken in sum

frequency of changes in occupational status as a consequence of SAH as found in various studies.

Apart from the differences in the frequency of limitations of occupational reintegration that exist between the individual studies and, in spite of the advances in treatment, between 20% and 60% of all patients after SAH cannot be reintegrated fully into professional life, also according to the more recent studies. In this respect, the incidence of decreased working capacity lies between 4% and 61% and the proportion of patients unable to work at 2–35%. This means that the large proportion of patients unable to work or restricted in working capacity by no means reflects the advances of medical management. Thus, in the era before microneurosurgery, in the study of Logue et al. (1968) a total of 44% of the patients had sustained occupational disadvantages due to SAH while, according to roughly comparable criteria, this figure still amounted to 31% in the study of Hütter, Gilsbach and Kreitschmann (1995). This raises a number of still unanswered questions as to the causes. Modern treatment methods might have lowered the mortality and morbidity of SAH patients considerably without having a positive influence on occupational reintegration. Last but not least, the possibility exists that neuropsychological rehabilitation in this patient group must still be tailored to the special requirements of this illness and be made more effective.

14. Neurobehavioral sequelae of SAH without a proven source of the bleeding in comparison to the sequelae of the rupture of an intracranial aneurysm

14.1. Comparison of the cognitive deficits in both patient groups

In 15–22% of all cases of non-traumatic spontaneous SAH a source of the bleeding cannot be identified even after repeated angiography (Cioffi et al., 1989; Alexander, Dias and Uttley, 1986; Spallone et al., 1986; Brismar and Sundbärg, 1985; Eskesen et al., 1984; Nishioka et al., 1984). Ferbert, Hubo and Biniek (1992) found in 38 of 91 patients after spontaneous non-traumatic SAH without a proven source of the bleeding (NA-SAH) a preponderant or exclusive distribution of blood in the prepontine and/or interpeduncular cistern. Ruelle et al. (1985) reported on an essentially more favorable course in 49 NA-SAH patients in comparison to patients after aneurysm rupture. Clinically relevant, angiographically proven vasospasm only occurred in 24.5% of the NA-SAH patients. Upon discharge only one patient presented with a hemiparesis and an aphasia (Ruelle et al., 1985). At follow-up 1–15 (median 8) years later, 94% of the patients were able to work to the same extent as before the hemorrhage.

In a series of studies, it could be shown, however, that also after NA-SAH many patients reported about complaints such as fatigue, forgetfulness, emotional changes, decreased tolerance toward strain and persisting headache. In some investigations, these complaints were approximately comparable to those of patients who had been operated after SAH due to aneurysm rupture (Hütter, Gilsbach and Kreitschmann, 1994; Oder et al., 1991; Ogden, Levin and Mee, 1990; Sonesson et al., 1989; Juul, Frediksen and Ringkjoeb, 1986; Shepard, 1984). Spallone et al. (1986) conducted a follow-up in 56 patients 2.6–15 years after NA-SAH with a good to fair neurological result (GOS = I–II). The authors found that half of their patients complained of frequent headache and cognitive slowing (Spallone et al., 1986). Sonesson et al. (1989) compared the neuropsychological test performance of 20 patients after NA-SAH and a good neurological result (GOS = I) with the test performance of SAH patients who had been operated upon. They found no significant differences between the two groups. This result stands in contradiction to the general opinion that NA-SAH exhibits a blander course and a more favorable long-term prognosis than SAH due to aneurysm rupture (Ferbert, Hubo and Biniek, 1992; Cioffi et al., 1989;

Alexander, Dias and Uttley, 1986; Brismar and Sundbärg, 1985; Nishioka et al., 1984). Eskesen et al. (1984) published data on the results of a follow-up of 42 NA-SAH patients exhibiting a good to fair neurological result (GOS = I–II). Three months to five years after the acute event, the patients were asked about their current problems and complaints either in a telephone interview or during a clinical follow-up. Complaints about headache and cognitive slowing were most often named in the study by Eskesen et al. (1984).

In a study by Hütter, Gilsbach and Kreitschmann (1994), 38 early operated patients and 20 patients after NA-SAH were investigated neuropsychologically one to five years after SAH. Between the two etiological groups comparable mean test scores and frequencies of cognitive deficits were found, whereby the patients in the operated group had sustained a significantly more severe bleeding (Fisher Grading). Also, a statistically non-significant trend for a worse clinical state (Hunt and Hess) was present in this group (Hütter, Gilsbach and Kreitschmann, 1994). Table 1 shows the results of the frequencies of cognitive deficits in both groups in the study by Hütter, Gilsbach and Kreitschmann (1994).

Table 1. Frequency of cognitive deficits in operated patients after SAH as compared to patients after SAH without proven source (NA-SAH)

Tests	Cognitive deficits				
	Aneurysm		NA-SAH		chi^2
	No.	%	No.	%	p
Token Test (aphasia)	9	23	1	5	0,409 ns
IQ-similarities	0	0	0	0	–
IQ-knowledge	0	0	0	0	–
IQ-pictures	0	0	0	0	–
IQ-mosaique	0	0	0	0	–
d2 speed	0	0	5	25	0,510 ns
d2 error %	1	2	2	10	0,974 ns
d2 error-reduced	0	0	7	35	0,669 ns
LPS-spatial think.	0	0	0	0	–
LPS-logical think.	0	0	0	0	–
IST-memory	6	15	6	30	0,710 ns
Benton test	10	26	12	60	0,717 ns
FWIT-interference	0	0	0	0	–
FWIT-selectivity	0	0	0	0	–
FWIT-wordfinding	0	0	0	0	–
Wiener errors[1]	6	15	9	45	0,397 ns
Wiener error %[1]	11	29	19	95	0,210 ns
Wiener corrects[1]	8	21	17	85	0,334 ns

[1]Wiener Determinationsgerät
ns = not significant
According to Hütter, Gilsbach and Kreitschmann (1994)

A comparison between clinically homogeneous subgroups who had sustained a comparably severe bleeding (Fisher > 1) and presented with a comparably poor state on admission to the clinic (Hunt and Hess > 2) revealed interesting results. The patients in the operated group were significantly more impaired in the area of short- and long-term memory and in word-finding capacity. The patients in the NA-SAH group again presented with significantly worse results in the areas of selectivity (FWIT subtest "interference") and in a complex choice reaction time task (Hütter, Gilsbach and Kreitschmann, 1994).

These results can be interpreted as evidence that the bleeding itself and associated pathophysiological processes constitute the main causes for the cognitive impairments after SAH, because on average no differences occurred. Provided that the severity of the bleeding was comparable, the NA-SAH patients were better in tests that are more likely to be sensitive to

Table 2. Means and standard deviations (SD) of the neuropsychological test performance of NA-SAH patients as compared to early operated patients 1–13 days after the hemorrhage

Tests	Aneurysm (n = 28)[a]		No aneurysm (n = 18)			
	Mean	SD	Mean	SD	t	p
Token Test[1] (errors)	3,6	5,2	2,2	3,5	0,86	0,39 ns
d2 concentration test speed[2]	96,8	10,8	101,7	22,6	0,97	0,33 ns
d2 concentration test error percent[2]	4,3	2,5	4,0	1,8	0,43	0,67 ns
d2 concentration testerror-reduced[2]	94,9	11,5	104,7	8,4	3,14	0,003*
IST-Memory[3](verbal long term memory)	90,6	7,5	96,1	9,8	2,07	0,04 ns
Benton[4] (no. Corrects)	5,0	2,2	5,3	2,1	0,31	0,71 ns
Reaction time[5]	298,4	109,2	287,5	60,2	0,37	0,71 ns
Alertness[5]	51,8	11,9	57,8	13,4	1,52	0,13 ns
Div. attention[5] (reaction time)	705,6	131,9	809,8	183,3	1,98	0,06 ns
Div. attention[5] (omissions)	4,0	3,8	4,0	3,9	0,05	0,96 ns
Go/NoGo task[5] (reaction time)	493,8	202,3	482,6	159,7	0,19	0,84 ns
Go/NoGo task[5] (errors)	39,8	13,9	48,6	17,2	1,85	0,07 ns

ns = not significant; $^{*}p < 0{,}01$; $^{**}p < 0{,}001$
[a]Early surgery (within 72 h)
[1]Aphasia screening-test: age-adjusted raw scores; [2]concentration test d2: standard values/stanine values; [3]verbal long-term memory: standard values; [4]short-term memory: No. correct reproductions; [5]Zimmermann testing battery: reaction times in milliseconds after age-correction; Alertness, errors in the Go/NoGo task: T-values; Div. = divided attention: No. of omissions; raw scores

Table 3. Cognitive functions tested, neuropsychological tests used and frequency of cognitive deficits after aneurysm rupture as compared to NA-SAH patients

Cognitive function	Neuropsycho-logical tests	Aneurysm rupture n=33 deficits[1]		NA-SAH group n=18 deficits[1]	
		No.	%	No.	%
Concentration speed	concentration test d2	4	12	0	–
Concentration error %	concentration test d2	13	39	5	28
Concentration error-reduced	concentration test d2	5	15	0	–
Aphasia screening	Token Test	9	27	3	17
Verbal long-term memory	IST Memory	18	55	6	33
Short term memory	Benton test	24	73	9	50
Simple reaction time	Zimmermann-testing battery[2]	8	27	5	30
Alertness	Zimmermann-testing battery[2]	2	7	0	–
Div. attention omissions[3]	Zimmermann-testing battery[2]	9	30	4	24
Div. attention reaction time[3]	Zimmermann-testing battery[2]	11	37	11	65
Go/NoGo task errors	Zimmermann-testing battery[2]	11	37	4	24
Go/NoGo task reaction time	Zimmermann-testing battery[2]	13	43	4	24

[1]Substantial cognitive deficit: performance 2 SD or more below the population mean according to the test norms; the Benton test and the Token test have cut-off scores for defining an individual deficit
[2]Because of technical difficulties with the testing computer the data of three patients in the group after aneurysmal SAH and of one patient after SAH of unknown origin have been lost
[3]Div. = divided; task for divided attention for the examination of the capacity of divided attention

focal brain damage than the operated patients. On the other hand, the NA-SAH patients showed poorer results in more unspecific tests more likely to be associated with general reaction capacity. This could be interpreted in such a way that in the operated patients focal deficits (such as aphasias) as a consequence of the intervention and/or due to a more malignant bleeding pattern superimpose on the unspecific ones which again are more prominent in the patients not operated upon. Here, again, a missing surgical removal of the subarachnoid blood could have had an unfavorable influence.

Not only in the chronic state after SAH but also in the acute stage a few days after the hemorrhage the average test results of both groups are comparable. In a study by Hütter, Kreitschmann-Andermahr and Gilsbach

Table 4. Neuropsychological impairments in patients after SAH without proven source of hemorrhage (NA-SAH) and in patients after aneurysm rupture

Authors	No.[1]	(Hunt & Hess)[2]	GOS Delay SAH/ Follow-up[3]	Non-aneurysmal SAH	Aneurysmal SAH
Spallone et al. (1986)	56	I–IV	I–II 2.6–15	50% headache 50% cognitive slowing	not examined
Eskesen et al. (1984)	42	I–IV	I–II 0.6–5	44% headache 41% cognitive slowing 29% reduced cognitive capacity 15% aphasia	not examined
Sonesson et al. (1989)	20	I–III	I 0.3–7	55% memory problems 33% reduced perceptual speed 33% reduced abstract thinking	56% memory problems 32% reduced perceptual speed 33% reduced abstract thinking
Ogden et al. (1990)	6	I–IV	I 5[b]	66% cognitive slowing 0% reduced mental flexibility 33% deficits long term memory 50% deficits short term memory 0% aphasia	20% cognitive slowing 50% reduced mental flexibility 40% deficits long term memory 40% deficits short term memory 10% aphasia
Hütter et al. (1994)	20	I–III	I–II 1–5	10–35% reduced concentration 30% deficits long term memory 60% impaired short term memory 45–95% slowing of reaction time 5% aphasia	2–4% reduced concentration 15% deficits long term memory 26% impaired short term memory 15–29% slowing of reaction time 23% aphasia
Hütter, Kreitschmann-Andermahr & Gilsbach (1998)	18	I–V	I–III 4[a]	0–28% reduced concentration 33% deficits long term memory 50% short term memory 24–65% disorders of attention 17% aphasia	12–39% reduced concentration 55% long term memory 73% short term memory 30–43% disorders of attention 27% aphasia

[a]Median
[b]Mean
[1]No. patients after SAH of unknown origin
[2]Neurological state on admission according to the grading of Hunt and Hess (1968)
[3]Neurological result according to the Glasgow Outcome Scale (GOS)/delay between SAH and follow-up examination in years

(1998) 51 patients between 2 and 13 (median12) days after SAH were investigated neuropsychologically a few days after the acute event. The study sample consisted of 28 early operated patients, 5 patients after late surgery and 18 patients without a proven source of the bleeding. The mean age was 57.7 years with a range between 26 and 65 years. There were 23 men and 28 women in the sample. Table 2 shows the comparison of mean test scores in the two groups. Table 3 gives an overview of the frequency and distribution of cognitive deficits between the two groups.

Regarding the neuropsychological effects of surgical aneurysm exclusion, it can be followed from these results that the intervention does, on average, not have additional damaging effects on the patient. This holds true at least under the prerequisite that the patients present with a good to fair neurological result upon discharge from inpatient treatment (Hütter, Kreitschmann-Andermahr and Gilsbach, 1998; Hütter and Gilsbach, 1996a). The worse performance in cognitive functions such as reaction time in the complex reaction choice task found by Hütter, Gilsbach and Kreitschmann (1994) in the NA-SAH patients in the chronic state, which is also reflected in poorer reaction time in a devided attention task in the acute state after SAH (Hütter, Kreitschmann-Andermahr and Gilsbach, 1998), are to be attributed to the hemorrhage itself and, possibly, to the missing surgical removal of the subarachnoid blood. The more frequent deficits in focal cognitive functions as aphasias in the operated patients could be explained by the higher incidence of intracerebral hemorrhages and, perhaps, by consequences of the intervention. Table 4 gives an overview of the results of studies on the neurobehavioral abnormalities in NA-SAH patients. The results of those studies are of special interest in which a direct comparison between NA-SAH patients and operated patients was undertaken.

Research conducted so far on the comparison of the cognitive deficits of NA-SAH and SAH due to aneurysm rupture reveals a number of methodological weaknesses. First, the group sizes are relatively small, especially in the NA-SAH patients. Therefore, the power of statistical tests to reveal significant differences is limited. On the other hand, no distinct differences can be expected, in the light of the previous results. Furthermore, in the majority of previous neuropsychological studies mostly NA-SAH patients treated in specialized neurosurgical departments have been included. It can be assumed, however, that especially those patients with severe bleedings are treated before all in neurosurgical centers. This selection bias should be taken into account in future studies.

14.2. Comparison of the impairments in quality of life between operated patients and those with SAH without a proven source of the bleeding

In the study of Hütter, Gilsbach and Kreitschmann (1995) patients after spontaneous non-traumatic SAH without a proven source of the bleeding (NA-SAH) did not only exhibit comparable impairments of their cognitive capacity as the operated patients but also in daily life and psychological adjustment. This result corresponds to earlier neuropsychological studies in which also no substantial differences in the frequency of cognitive impairments and emotional changes between the two groups were found (Hütter, 1998; Hütter, Gilsbach and Kreitschmann, 1995; 1994; Ogden, Mee and Henning, 1993a; Ogden, Levin and Mee, 1990; Sonesson et al., 1989). In the study of Ogden, Levin and Mee (1990) the authors compared 10 patients with a ruptured and operated aneurysm and a very small group of six patients after NA-SAH. They found that the ability to work was significantly more often reduced in the latter group. The NA-SAH patients were also stressed by more pronounced fatigue and were more impaired in their free-time activities. Among the operated patients, 10% with clinically relevant depression were found whereas among the NA-SAH patients 50% exhibited a clinically relevant depressive disorder (Ogden, Levin and Mee, 1990). An increased level of anxiety was found, in tendency, more frequently in the

Table 5. Means and standard deviations (SD) of the ALQI proxy- and self-rating version subscales in the group of the operated patients and the NA-SAH patients

	Aneurysmal SAH (n = 29)		SAH of unknown origin (n = 16)			
ALQI subscales+	Self-rating	Proxy-rating[2]	Self-rating	Proxy-rating[2]	t-test Self-rating	t-test Proxy-rating
Activation	2,4 (2,5)	2,6 (2,7)	2,8 (2,3)	4,0 (2,8)	p = 0,05 ns	p = 0,00[1]
Mobility	0,9 (1,4)	0,9 (1,6)	0,6 (1,0)	0,6 (1,0)	p = 0,05 ns	p = 0,05 ns
House-work	2,0 (2,4)	2,7 (3,0)	2,0 (1,8)	3,0 (2,5)	p = 0,09 ns	p = 0,07 ns
Social contact	2,9 (2,5)	3,2 (2,8)	2,1 (1,9)	3,6 (3,0)	p = 0,03 ns	p = 0,06 ns
Family relations	1,5 (1,8)	1,8 (1,9)	1,0 (1,6)	2,6 (2,9)	p = 0,03 ns	p = 0,03 ns
Free-time activities	3,3 (2,8)	3,9 (2,6)	2,4 (2,4)	3,2 (2,1)	p = 0,02 ns	p = 0,03 ns
Ambulation	1,6 (1,8)	1,5 (1,6)	1,6 (1,9)	2,0 (1,8)	p = 0,09 ns	p = 0,03 ns
Communication	1,0 (1,7)	1,1 (1,8)	0,1 (0,5)	0,6 (1,0)	p = 0,00[1]	p = 0,03 ns
Autonomy	0,1 (0,4)	0,0 (0,1)	0,0 (0,0)	0,0 (0,0)	p = 0,01 ns	p = 0,04 ns
Cognition	6,8 (4,9)	7,6 (4,4)	4,8 (2,9)	7,0 (4,0)	p = 0,00 ns	p = 0,06 ns
ALQI Total score	22,7 (18,6)	25,5 (18,3)	17,9 (11,6)	26,6 (16,9)	p = 0,03 ns	p = 0,08 ns
ALQI Psycho-social score	11,2 (10,0)	12,7 (10,0)	8,7 (6,7)	14,0 (10,0)	p = 0,03 ns	p = 0,07 ns
ALQI Physical score	4,7 (5,5)	5,1 (5,4)	4,3 (3,6)	5,6 (4,4)	p = 0,08 ns	p = 0,07 ns

ns = not significant; $^{*}p < 0,05$; $^{**}p < 0,001$

[1]The ALQI subscale "work" was not included because only 19 patients worked regularly

[2]The partner-ratings were based on the data of 27 life companions of the patients after aneurysm rupture and of 13 partners of NA-SAH patients

NA-SAH patients (50%) than in the operated patients (40%). Also in a later study, Ogden, Mee and Henning (1993a) found in a structured interview pertaining to psychosocial adjustment and including the life-companions of the patients, no significant differences with respect to general impairments between operated and NA-SAH patients. Moreover, the NA-SAH patients were more impaired in the areas of work and free-time activities and reported of significantly more problems with increased tiredness (Ogden, Mee and Henning, 1993a). Possibly, this increased tiredness is also the consequence of the perimesencephalic bleeding pattern frequently observed in NA-SAH (van Gijn et al., 1985b), since Hütter, Kreitschmann-Andermahr and Gilsbach (1998) were able to show that substantial impairments in reaction time in a divided reaction task were found in this patient group due to brainstem damage. This result supports the hypothesis that NA-SAH patients are especially impaired in diffuse cognitive functions as initiative and attention capacity which can possibly be interpreted as a direct consequence of the bleeding.

So far no investigation pertaining to health-related quality of life in the two patient groups has been conducted using a standardized procedure. Therefore, in an own study, 45 patients and their life-companions were investigated with respect to their impairments in daily life by means of the Aachen Life Quality Inventory (ALQI) in order to perform a comparison between NA-SAH and operated patients. The mean age was 47 years with a range between 30 and 69 years. The study sample consisted of 20 men and 25 women after spontaneous non-traumatic SAH, 29 of whom had been operated upon early whereas in 16 patients no source of the bleeding could be established. Table 5 gives an overview of all results of the comparison of health-related quality of life in the two patient groups.

The only statistically significant difference in self-rated quality of life between the two groups emerged in the ALQI subscale "Communication" where the operated patients reported of significantly ($p < 0.05$) more impairments. The life-companions again rated the patients in the NA-SAH group as significantly ($p = 0.04$) more impaired in the area of activation as compared to the operated patients. Here, in concurrence with earlier findings, it becomes evident that in the functions of initiative and activation at least in the perspective of the patients' partners a more pronounced impairment of the NA-SAH patients emerged. The operated patients rated themselves as more impaired in more "focal" functions, i.e. in the area of communication. This result corresponds exactly to the neuropsychological findings where the NA-SAH patients showed a more pronounced cognitive slowing in the acute stage of the illness whereas patients after aneurysm rupture rather presented with focal cognitive deficits such as aphasias (Hütter, Kreitschmann-Andermahr and Gilsbach, 1998; Hütter, Gilsbach and Kreitschmann, 1995; 1994). At present, the question remains open whether these different patterns of neuropsychological impairments can be traced back to differences in the bleeding pattern, the surgical intervention or a combination of both variables in the two groups.

15. Neuropsychological sequelae of aneurysm surgery

At present only few studies on the direct neuropsychological sequelae of operative measures and events in aneurysm surgery have been published. This shortcoming is all the more serious before the background that an increasing number of authors recently found no significant influence of different aneurysm locations on neuropsychological test performance (Hütter and Gilsbach, 1996a; 1995a; 1992; Hütter, Gilsbach and Kreitschmann, 1995; Tidswell et al., 1995; Satzger et al., 1995; Ogden, Mee and Henning, 1993a; DeLuca, 1993; 1992a;b; Richardson, 1991; 1989; DeLuca and Cicerone, 1991; Vilkki et al., 1989). Therefore, the surgical exclusion of a ruptured intracranial aneurysm as a possible cause of the observed neuropsychological abnormalities moves further into the foreground. Evidence for a potentially damaging effect of aneurysm surgery even under microneurosurgical conditions is provided by the study of Hornyak, Gilsbach and Harders (1991), who found that of the 23 patients in their consecutive series exhibiting postoperative infarcts, these could be attributed in 19 (83%) patients most probably to the surgical intervention. Prolonged temporary clipping as well as inadvertent damage to vessels or vascular occlusions, respectively, were named by the authors as possible causes (Hornyak, Gilsbach and Harders, 1991). These results imply that even modern microneurosurgical aneurysm surgery can be associated with an appreciable risk of damage to the patient.

For a long time, the neuropsychological sequelae of different surgical procedures, intraoperative complications and associated events remained unclear. One neuroanatomically well-founded result consists therein that prudent clipping of ACoA aneurysms with special attention to the perforators emanating from the ACoA and the A1 segment prevents the emergence of massive memory disturbances and/or psychopathological syndromes such as Korsakoff syndrome (Hütter and Gilsbach, 1996a; 1992; Gade, 1982). Results on the significance of different surgical techniques in aneurysm surgery especially in regard of the neuropsychological sequelae in patients with ruptured ACoA aneurysms has been published already in 1982 by A. Gade (Gade, 1982). The author found a clear relationship between the intraoperative ligature of the ACoA and postoperative memory deficits up to amnesias and Korsakoff syndromes. When an ACoA aneurysm in the study by Gade (1982) had been excluded by means of the trapping procedure, in nine (81%) of 11 patients a postoperative amnestic syndrome emerged, whereas only six (16%) of 37 patients exhibited a postoperative amnestic syndrome when the neck of the aneurysm had been clipped (Gade, 1982). This result can be explained in such a way that the operating microscope and modern microneurosurgical removable aneurysm clips allow a careful exclusion of the aneurysm without damage to the parent vessel itself or the small perforators emanating from the ACoA (Hütter and Gilsbach, 1996a; 1992; Gilsbach et al., 1988a; Gilsbach and Harders, 1989; Gilsbach, 1988; Yasargil, 1984; Gade, 1982; Yasargil, Fox and Ray, 1975). The consequent use of the operating microscope and modern removable aneurysm clips make it easier for the neurosurgeon to prevent damage to the small perforating vessels originating from the ACoA which supply subcallosal areas at the anterior wall of the third ventricle and especially the nucleus basalis Meynert. Yasargil, Fox and Ray (1975) reported that of 203 operated aneurysms of the ACoA, eight (3.9%) patients developed a persisting psychoorganic syndrome postoperatively, consisting of confusion, disorientation, dementia and lack of initiative. Interestingly, of these patients, four had been operated using the trapping procedure (Yasargil, Fox and Ray, 1975). On the other side, Richardson (1991) found no difference between those patients in whom the aneurysm had been clipped and those in whom the aneurysm had been excluded by means of ligature of the carotid artery. Mercier et al. (1991) reported that the neuropsychological impairments of their patients were also dependent on the qualification of their surgeon. Unfortunately, details on this result are missing in the study of Mercier et al. (1991).

Maurice-Williams et al. (1991) investigated 27 patients after aneurysm rupture in a prospective study with one preoperative and two follow-up investigations on the day of discharge from inpatient treatment and one year later. All patients had been operated upon late without any surgical complications having occurred. Temporary occlusion of a vessel proximal of the aneurysm had not been required in any case. At the time of the first postoperative follow-up, the test performance in 11 (41%) patients had become substantially worse as compared to the preoperative investigation and one patient exhibited a new aphasia. Persisting deficits were explained by the authors by prolonged intraoperative ischemia, prolonged retraction of the dominant hemisphere and inadvertent occlusion of the right anterior choriodal artery in one patient (Maurice-Williams et al., 1991). The authors were not able to find a relationship between postoperative test performance and the extent of induced hypotension or intraoperative aneurysm rupture (Maurice-Williams et al., 1991).

The results of several studies where patients after spontaneous nontraumatic SAH without a proven source of the bleeding exhibited comparable cognitive deficits as the operated patients speak against a general harmful effect of aneurysm surgery (Hütter, Kreitschmann-Andermahr and Gilsbach, 1998; Hütter, Gilsbach and Kreitschmann, 1994; Sonesson et al., 1989). In a study by Hütter and Gilsbach (1996a), a consecutive series of 28 patients was investigated neuropsychologically between one and 13 days (median 5 days) after early surgery (within 72 hours) of a ruptured intracranial aneurysm. In a further still unpublished study, 45 of these patients could be followed-up four years later with respect to their HRQOL using the Aachen Life Quality Inventory (ALQI). Plegias, other severe neurological impairments, fluent aphasias or acute psychoses were exclusion criteria. The neurological result of all patients was estimated as good six months after discharge from acute inpatient treatment (GOS = I). Induced hypotension had not been used during a single intervention. Neither a significantly unfavorable effect of premature intraoperative aneurysm rupture nor of the side of surgical approach (left versus right peritonal) on neuropsychological test performance in the acute stage of the illness and on later quality of life was found. Also Heiskanen and Vilkki (1981) could establish no effect of side (left versus right) of surgical approach in 25 patients between six months and 11 years after the intervention.

In the study by Hütter and Gilsbach (1996a), temporary clipping of vessels was unavoidable in 18 (64%) operations. The mean time of temporary clipping was 2.8 minutes with a range between two and 13 minutes. In those patients in whom temporary clipping was unavoidable, test performance in the concentration test d2 and an alertness task (Zimmermann testing battery) was significantly poorer than in the patients in whom intraoperatively no temporary clipping of vessels had been used ($p < 0.05$, respectively). Four years later the patients in whom temporary clipping of a vessel had been necessary rated themselves as significantly more impaired in the ALQI subscale "Mobility" ($p = 0.05$). On the other hand, it cannot be excluded that complicating factors such as generally difficult surgery, sudden fall of blood pressure or individual collateralization could have confounded the persisting unfavorable effects of temporary clipping. Tidswell et al. (1995) reported that temporary clipping of the ACA was associated with a significantly higher impairment in daily life, according to the assessment of the life-companions of the patients. Moreover, in an individual patient with a PCoA aneurysm in whom temporary clipping of the vessel had been inavoidable, immediately postoperatively a severe deficit in verbal memory performance emerged (Tidswell et al., 1995). The risk associated with temporary clipping of vessels in aneurysm surgery is a matter of debate among neurosurgeons (Samson et al., 1994; Charbel et al., 1991; Schramm et al., 1990; Seifert et al., 1989a; Wassmann, Werner and Stockert, 1989; Jabre and Symon, 1987; Batjer and Samson, 1986; Perneczky and Koos, 1982). Nevertheless, the present standard of knowledge is not sufficient to predict the tolerance of temporary clipping reliably for every patient and each vessel (Schramm et al., 1990). Despite all methodological difficulties this would be a desired aim for future clinical studies.

Resection of parts of the gyrus rectus was associated in the study of Hütter and Gilsbach (1996a) in the acute stage of the illness with a median of five days after surgery with a significantly worse performance in short-term memory. Further statistical analyses excluded a confounding effect of ACoA aneurysm location (Hütter and Gilsbach, 1996a). On the other hand, at the time of follow-up four years later no persisting unfavorable effects of the resection of parts of the gyrus rectus on quality or life of the patients could be established. In ACoA patients in whom the gyrus rectus had been resected, Teissier du Cros and Lhermitte (1984) found between 12 and 50 months after aneurysm surgery a significantly worse Wechsler memory quotient in comparison to those ACoA patients in whom this operative measure had not been necessary. According to anatomical-morphological, hodological and functional studies, it can be expected that the gyrus rectus is the anatomical extension of the cingulate gyrus (Morecraft, Geula and Mesulam, 1992; Pardo et al., 1990; Pandya, van Hoesen and Mesulam, 1981). The enormous functional and especially neuropsychological relevance of the gyrus cinguli has been verified by an increasing number of studies published within the last years (Devinsky, Morrell and Vogt, 1995).

The timing of aneurysm surgery is matter of intensive discussion among neurosurgeons. The supporters of late surgery bring forward that the surgical risk and the probability to induce additional damage to the patient by the intervention is larger during early surgery, since the brain is more vulnerable immediately after the hemorrhage. Those in favor of early surgery allege that the surgical risk is not higher but that the patient is spared the risk of fatal rebleeding because of the early exclusion of the aneurysm. Satzger et al. (1995) compared 22 early operated (within 72 hours) to 22 late operated patients with respect to the degree of cognitive impairments, assessed by means of an extensive neuropsychological test battery. No significant differences between both groups were found (Satzger et al., 1995). Also Sonesson et al. (1987) were not able to establish an unfavorable effect of early surgery on cognitive performance capacity of their patients. Both groups were comparable regarding their neuropsychological test performance (Sonesson et al., 1987).

In the last 10 years, a new minimal invasive procedure, endovascular occlusion of ruptured as well as innocent intracranial aneurysms by means of metal coils was developed as an alternative to microneurosurgical clipping (Guglielmi et al., 1991; Hodes et al., 1991). A major argument for the endovascular procedures lies in the avoidance of surgical mortality and morbidity associated with an intracranial surgical intervention. In view of the neurological result (GOS), the endovascular method shows a comparable risk for causing neurological deficits as the surgical exclusion of an intracranial aneurysm (Spetzger et al., 1997;1996; Spetzger, Rohde and Gilsbach, 1997). Tooth et al. (1997) compared the neuropsychological result of 15 patients treated by means of endovascular coiling with a control group of patients whose aneurysms had been clipped microneurosurgically. Furthermore, an MRI was performed for the investigation of morphological damage. In the operated patients substantially more structural damage that could be put down largely to the consequences of the intervention was seen than in the patients treated by endovascular coiling. On the other hand no difference in neuropsychological test performance between the two groups was found. This led Tooth et al. (1997) to the conclusion that the endovascular treatment method did not ameliorate the neuropsychological result of patients substantially one year after aneurysm rupture. The findings of Tooth et al. (1997) can also be interpreted in such a way that the hemorrhage as the underlying real illness remains untreated by means of the endovascular method. By this way, secondary complications can lead to or worsen neuropsychological impairments. Even if the surgical intervention leads to more morphological brain damage, this effect might be compensated for by the intraoperative removal of subarachnoid blood and blood clots and the resulting prevention of secondary complications, in contrast to the untreated hemorrhage in the case of coiling.

The data available so far supply some evidence that inadequate clipping of aneurysms, temporary clipping of perforating vessels, prolonged retraction of the brain and operative damage to vessels or brain parenchyma constitute an appreciable risk to damage the patient additionally and thus to cause persisting neurobehavioral impairments. The results of the study by Hütter and Gilsbach (1996a) in so far underestimate the risk of the surgical intervention since the data are based on a selected patient sample all of whom could be investigated neuropsychologically in the acute stage of their illness and who exhibited without exception already at discharge a good neurological result (GOS = I). It can, therefore, not be excluded that the patients damaged substantially due to the intervention were not included in the study sample of Hütter and Gilsbach (1996a).

16. Neurobehavioral sequelae of the anatomical bleeding pattern

Several authors stress the great prognostic relevance of the presence of intraventricular and/or intracerebral blood for the neurological result after SAH, even if the amount of further subarachnoid blood is small (Gerber et al., 1993; Auer, Schneider and Auer, 1986; Adams, Kassell and Torner, 1985; Gurusinghe and Richardson, 1984; Fisher, Kistler and Davis, 1980). From a neuropsychological point of view, Odgen, Mee and Henning (1993a) reported that SAH patients with intracerebral hemorrhage exhibited a significantly worse memory performance 10 weeks after the acute event which persisted at follow-up 12 months later. However, Tidswell et al. (1995) could not find any correlation between the bleeding pattern on CCT and the cognitive deficits of the patients. It does not become clear from the study of Tidswell et al. (1995) according to which criteria the CCT scans had been evaluated and which aspects of the bleeding pattern were investigated by the authors.

It was the aim of a study by Hütter, Kreitschmann-Andermahr and Gilsbach (1998) to elucidate whether substantial correlations between neuropsychological test performance and the anatomical pattern of the bleeding existed in patients after SAH. The original hypothesis of Hütter, Kreitschmann-Andermahr and Gilsbach (1998) was that specific effects of the bleeding pattern would be most pronounced in the first days after the bleeding and, therefore, would exert its most prominent neuropsychological effect at that early stage. A consecutive series of 51 patients not older than 65 years was, therefore, investigated in the study of Hütter, Kreitschmann-Andermahr and Gilsbach (1998) 1–13 (median 4) days after SAH by means of a number of neuropsychological tests. Of the 51 patients in the study sample 33 had been operated upon, in 28 of them early surgery within 72 hours had been possible. The remaining 18 patients had sustained spontaneous non-traumatic SAH without a proven source of the bleeding. The neurological result at six-month follow-up ranged from GOS = I to GOS = III. In a further own study, a follow-up four years later on health-related quality of life could be conducted in 45 (88%) of these patients.

Frontal intracerebral hemorrhage according to CCT was diagnosed in the acute stage in 8 (16%) patients. In the acute stage of the illness these patients exhibited a highly significant poorer test performance as compared to all other SAH patients in the aphasia screening test ($p < 0.000$), in simple reaction time ($p < 0.000$) and in the Go/NoGo task ($p < 0.000$). At the time of the four-year follow-up, patients with frontal intracerebral hemorrhage showed significantly more impairments in the areas of activation ($p = 0.04$) and housework ($p = 0.03$) as well as in the ALQI Physical sum score ($p = 0.03$). A distribution of blood with accentuation in the right carotid cistern, ambient cistern, cisterna cruralis or sylvii was ascertained in 6 (12%) patients according to the initial CCT. These patients made significantly ($p < 0.01$) less errors in the aphasia screening test (Token Test). At follow-up four years later, they rated themselves as significantly less impaired in the quality of life area "Communication" ($p = 0.01$).

Intraventricular hemorrhage (IVH) was diagnosed by means of CCT in 13 (25%) patients. Five of these patients, however, exhibited acute hydrocephalus at the time of neuropsychological investigation. In order to investigate a possible interaction between the two variables, a 2×2 analysis of variance with the factors hydrocephalus and presence of intraventricular blood was calculated. The presence of intraventricular blood showed an exclusive unfavorable main effect on the accuracy of concentration capacity ($p = 0.001$), error-reduced concentration capacity ($p < 0.01$), reaction time ($p = 0.007$) and omissions ($p < 0.01$) in a divided attention task. The frequency of errors in the Go/NoGo task was explained by the presence of intraventricular blood ($p < 0.01$) and acute hydrocephalus ($p < 0.01$) which formed significant main effects without the occurrence of an interaction. Moreover, a significant main effect of acute hydrocephalus ($p = 0.016$) was found in the Go/NoGo task regarding reaction time. Furthermore, a significant interaction between hydrocephalus and IVH with respect to reaction time in the Go/NoGo task ($p < 0.01$) occurred.

In order to control statistically the possibility that the long-term effects of IVH on quality of life were confounded with the late effects of hydrocephalus in the acute stage of the illness four years ago, 2×2 analyses of variance were calculated with the factors hydrocephalus and IVH. Significant main effects of acute hydrocephalus on the area "Activation" of self-rated quality of life ($p = 0.05$) and IVH on the extent of impairment in the ALQI subscale "Family relations" ($p = 0.03$) were found. Significant main effects of IVH were seen regarding the ALQI subscales "Mobility" ($p < 0.05$), "Family relations" ($p = 0.02$) and "Ambulation" ($p = 0.01$) according to proxy-rating. By the assessment of the life-companions, those patients in whom acute hydrocephalus had occurred exhibited significantly more impairments in the areas of "Activation" ($p = 0.05$) and "Housework" ($p = 0.02$). Furthermore, a significant interaction between IVH and hydrocephalus ($p = 0.001$) was found regarding impairments in the ALQI subscale "Mobility".

It can be concluded from these results that the neurobehavioral sequelae of IVH are independent of disturbed CSF circulation and exhibit a permanent compromising effect on health-related quality of life. The breakthrough of blood associated with IVH predominantly through frontal brain parenchyma (area subcallosa, hypothalamus, septum pellucidum as well as parts of the internal capsule; compare Fig. 1, chapter 4) and mechanical damage to paraventricular structures (Mayfrank, 1997), should probably be the cause for the neurobehavioral impairments especially in areas of motor function. Frontal intracerebral hemorrhage shows specific and pronounced effects on those cognitive functions as perseveration tendency and simple reaction time, typically regarded as sequelae of frontal brain damage (Hütter, 1997a;b). This also holds true for some areas of the life quality registered four years later. Therefore, the psychosocial adjustment disturbances, observed frequently after SAH can also be put down to latent frontal brain damage. This damage must not be necessarily be visible on CCT or MRI. Such an interpretation is underlined by the fact that in the own study sample only two patients exhibited manifest frontal brain damage on late CCT (six months after the acute event) such as infarction or hypodensities.

17. Short- and long-term effects of disturbed CSF circulation after SAH

Despite the meanwhile routine use of CCT in patients with SAH, effects of disturbances of the circulation of cerebrospinal fluid (CSF) have rarely been investigated scientifically in patients after SAH. Vassilouthis and Richardson (1979) saw no clinical problem in ventricular enlargement after SAH. On the other hand, Menon, Weir and Overton (1981) observed a decreased cerebral blood flow (CBF) and a poorer clinical state in patients with ventricular enlargement in the acute state after SAH. Hydrocephalus in the acute stage after SAH seems to constitute a particularly unfavorable prognostic factor (Mohr et al., 1983). Van Gijn et al. (1985a) reported that in 30 of 34 patients with acute hydrocephalus after SAH a substantially deteriorated state of consciousness was observed. Hütter, Gilsbach and Kreitschmann (1995) found that, one to four years after SAH according to the assessment of the life-companions, those patients who had developed hydrocephalus in the postacute clinical course and in whom shunt insertion had been performed were still significantly more impaired in daily life than the patients who had not developed hydrocephalus.

Accordingly, in a further study with 45 patients after SAH, Hütter (1998) found that those who had developed hydrocephalus in the postacute course treated by shunt insertion were significantly ($p = 0.04$) more impaired by subjective strain (FPI-R) than patients without this secondary complication. Odgen, Mee and Henning (1993a) reported that the presence of hydrocephalus was associated with a poorer performance in memory tests in the postacute stage and 10 weeks after SAH. However, at a further follow-up one year later no difference was observed anymore (Odgen, Mee and Henning, 1993a). On the other hand, Laiacona et al. (1989) could not find any correlation between enlarged ventricles and the cognitive impairments of patients after aneurysm rupture. In the study by Hütter, Kreitschmann-Andermahr and Gilsbach (1998) with 51 patients in the acute state after SAH (1–13 days after the hemorrhage or surgery, respectively), even transient disturbances of CSF circulation, which did not reach the extent of acute hydrocephalus and were treated by means of daily lumbar puncture, had measurable neuropsychological sequelae. In these patients performance in long-term memory was significantly ($p < 0.01$) worse than in the other patients.

Acute hydrocephalus was diagnosed in 13 (25%) patients in the study sample of Hütter, Kreitschmann-Andermahr and Gilsbach (1998). Of these, eight were treated by means of at least daily repeated lumbar puncture whereas in the other patients transient lumbar drainage was performed. These patients exhibited a significantly worse long-term memory ($p < 0.001$), a slower simple reaction time ($p < 0.1$) and made significantly more errors in the Go/NoGo task ($p = 0.002$) than the patients without acute hydrocephalus. Of these 51 patients 45 (88%) could be investigated in an own still unpublished study regarding their health-related quality of life four years after the acute event. Mean age was 47 years with a range between 30 and 69 years. There were 20 men and 25 women in the study sample after spontaneous non-traumatic SAH, 29 of whom had been operated upon mostly early whereas no source of the bleeding could be proven in 16 patients. Table 38 shows the comparison of the mean scores in the ALQI subscales and the sum scores of the self- as well as proxy-rated quality of life between the 10 patients presenting with a disturbance of CSF circulation below the threshold of acute hydrocephalus and the 35 patients without this complication in the acute state after the hemorrhage.

Those patients who had developed a subacute disturbance of CSF circulation in the acute stage of the illness after SAH rated themselves four years later as significantly ($p = 0.01$) more impaired in the ALQI subscale "Activation" (Table 1). In the perspective of the life-partners, these differences were even more pronounced. Thus, substantially more impairments in the life quality areas of "Activation" ($p = 0.01$), "House-work" ($p < 0.01$), "Social contact" ($p < 0.05$) and "Family relations" ($p < 0.01$) were registered in patients with a disturbance of CSF circulation in the acute stage after SAH (Table 1). According to the assessments by the life-companions, these patients exhibited significantly more impairments in the ALQI Psycho-Social score of the ALQI summary scores.

Of the 45 patients whose data had been available at the time of follow-up, 12 (27%) had developed hydrocephalus within one year after the acute event which was treated in all of them by permanent shunt insertion. These patients rated themselves at the time of follow-up as significantly ($p = 0.02$) more impaired in the ALQI subscale "Cognition" than those patients without hydrocephalus. The severity of the bleeding according to CCT criteria (Fisher Score) and the neurological state on admission (Hunt and Hess) were comparable between both groups. This implies that possibly not all neuropsychological sequelae of hydrocephalus can be compensated by shunt insertion (Hütter, Mayfrank and Gilsbach, submitted). The neuropsychological sequelae of disturbed CSF circulation in adults, the effects of various treatment methods and possible late consequences as well as their causes have so far only been investigated infrequently in neuropsychological research. Hardemark et al. (1989) could not establish any correlation between hypodensities or infarcts, respectively, on a late CCT and the results of neuropsychological assessment two years after SAH, but substantial associations between the extent of abnormal ventricular enlargement and neuropsychological test performance occurred (Hardemark et al., 1989).

Table 1. Means and standard deviations (SD) in the ALQI subscales of patients with disturbances of the circulation of cerebrospinal fluid (CSF) and in patients without a disturbance of the CSF circulation

	No disturbance of CSF circulation (n = 35)		Disturbance of CSF circulation (n = 10)			
ALQI subscales+	self-rating	proxy-rating[2]	self-rating	proxy-rating[2]	t-test self-rating	t-test proxy-rating
Activation	2,1 (2,3)	2,5 (2,5)	4,3 (2,1)	5,0 (2,7)	0,01[1]	0,01[1]
Movement	0,8 (1,3)	0,7 (1,3)	0,6 (1,3)	1,1 (1,9)	0,56 ns	0,54 ns
House-work	1,9 (2,0)	2,1 (2,4)	2,8 (2,6)	4,9 (3,3)	0,26 ns	0,009[1]
Social contact	2,5 (2,5)	2,8 (2,5)	3,3 (1,8)	5,2 (3,0)	0,39 ns	0,02 [1]
Family relations	1,2 (1,9)	1,5 (2,0)	1,8 (0,9)	3,7 (2,4)	0,42 ns	0,009[1]
Free-time activities	2,9 (2,7)	3,4 (2,5)	3,5 (3,3)	4,7 (2,3)	0,55 ns	0,18 ns
Ambulation	1,6 (1,7)	1,7 (1,8)	1,8 (1,5)	1,4 (1,3)	0,53 ns	0,53 ns
Communication	0,7 (1,6)	1,0 (1,7)	0,7 (1,0)	0,9 (0,9)	0,94 ns	0,86 ns
Autonomy	0,8 (0,3)	0,3 (0,1)	0,0 (0,0)	0,0 (0,0)	0,46 ns	0,56 ns
Cognition	5,9 (4,4)	7,2 (4,3)	7,0 (4,3)	8,5 (4,0)	0,50 ns	0,41 ns
ALQI Total score	20,1 (17,1)	23,3 (16,8)	25,8 (14,2)	35,4 (17,3)	0,34 ns	0,06 ns
ALQI Psycho-social score	9,6 (9,4)	11,4 (9,7)	13,6 (6,8)	19,8 (8,7)	0,23 ns	0,02[1]
ALQI Physical score	4,5 (4,9)	4,7 (4,6)	5,2 (4,8)	7,4 (6,0)	0,72 ns	0,16 ns

ns = not significant; * $p < 0,05$; ** $p < 0,001$

[1]The ALQI subscale "Work" could not be included because only 19 patients worked regularly

[2]The results of the proxy-ratings are based on the data of 30 life companions of patients without any indication for a disturbed CSF circulation and of 10 life companions of patients who exhibited a disturbed CSF circulation but not corresponding to an acute hydrocephalus

18. Health-related quality of life in patients who had been in Hunt and Hess grades IV or V on admission to the neurosurgical unit

Next to a substantial reduction of mortality and morbidity, the progress that has modified neurosurgical treatment of ruptured intracranial aneurysms considerably in the last years has led to increasingly frequent surgery on patients in Hunt and Hess grades IV or V on admission to the neurosurgical unit. In some centers, it is attempted to attain an exclusion of the ruptured aneurysm by early surgery in all patients in a Hunt and Hess grade IV or V with only few exceptions (Hütter et al., 1998; LeRoux et al., 1996b; Spetzger and Gilsbach, 1994; Seifert, Trost and Stolke, 1990; Bailes et al., 1990; Gilsbach et al., 1989; 1988b; Brandt et al., 1987). On the basis of the poor prognosis in this group of SAH patients the question arises in how far and under what conditions the patients surviving after maximal medical therapy show an acceptable quality of life in their later everyday life. Therefore, verification of the prognostic relevance of a number of clinical variables is important for the later quality of life. For this reason, at the Department of Neurosurgery of the University Hospital of the University of Technology (RWTH) Aachen, a prospective study was conducted with the intent to contribute to the clarification of the open questions associated herewith. A consecutive series of 192 patients who had been operated upon a ruptured aneurysm between 1990 and June 1992 in the Departments of Neurosurgery of the RWTH Aachen were investigated with regard to their HRQOL 2–3 years after the acute event using the ALQI (Hütter and Gilsbach, 1996b; 1995b). Of these 39 (20.3%) patients had been in a clinical state grade IV or V after Hunt and Hess on admission to the unit, whereas 153 were in a clinical state grade I–III according to Hunt and Hess. In the group of patients with grades IV or V, 33 (84.6%) patients were operated upon early (within 72 hours). In the Hunt and Hess group IV or V, 12 (30.7) died during the acute stage of their illness while a further 5 (12.8%) had died until follow-up two to three years after discharge. In the patient group in a more favorable clinical state on admission to the unit, six (3.9) died during the acute stage of their illness while a further 10 (6.5) patients had died until follow-up.

Therefore, data on HRQOL of 119 patients were available at follow-up. The self-rated quality of life of the surviving patients in Hunt and Hess grades IV or V on admission to the unit (n = 20) was significantly more impaired in the life quality areas ambulation, mobility, social contact, freetime-activities, communication, autonomy and cognitive capacity ($p < 0.05$, respectively) as compared to the patients in a clinical state I–III ($n = 99$). Age, number and severity of accompanying illnesses and sociodemographic variables were comparable between both groups. A detailed analysis of the quality of life in the group with a worse initial clinical state (Hunt and Hess IV or V) revealed that only six (30%) patients enjoyed a good to acceptable quality of life, defined according to the upper quarter of the study sample. Statistical analyses revealed no significant differences between these two groups in terms of mean blood flow velocity (TCD), aneurysm location, number and severity of accompanying illnesses, delay SAH/surgery, severity of the bleeding (Fisher Score), incidence of intracerebral or intraventricular hemorrhages or hydrocephalus. However, with a mean age of 42.2 years, the patients in the group with an acceptable quality of life were significantly ($p = 0.006$) younger than the other patients with a mean age of 54.9 years. By means of a discriminant analysis, 85% of the patients initially in a clinical state grade IV or V after Hunt and Hess could be classified correctly as belonging to the group with an acceptable quality of life or the impaired patients, respectively. Patient age proved to be the only discriminating variable. This implies that age is an important predictor of later quality of life also in patients in an initial state grade IV or V after Hunt and Hess. Younger patients who were in a clinical state grades IV or V after Hunt and Hess after the rupture of an intracranial aneurysm on admission to the unit and were operated upon early afterwards have a realistic chance to regain a later good to acceptable HRQOL. However, these results, especially those of the multivariate analysis, must be interpreted with caution since the number of cases in the individual subgroups of patients in an initially poor neurological state is still relatively small. But also in other studies, age proved an important prognostic predictor of mortality and morbidity after aneurysm rupture (Lanziano et al., 1996; LeRoux et al., 1996b; Deruty et al., 1995; Gilsbach and Harders, 1989; Gilsbach et al., 1988b).

19. Vasospasm: a risk factor for neuropsychological impairments after SAH?

Richardson (1989) found a significantly unfavorable influence of severe angiographically proven postoperative vasospasm on memory performance in comparison to those patients with no or only slight vasospasm. In a retrospective study of 219 patients two to 14 years after SAH, Larsson et al. (1989) found no influence of angiographically proven vasospasm in the acute stage of the illness on later neuropsychological test performance in working memory (Larsson et al., 1989). On the other hand, Gade (1982) found that in amnestics angiographically proven vasospasm was present in the acute stage more frequently, while, in contrast, Teissier Du Cros and Lhermitte (1984) were not able to demonstrate such a connection. In the study of Stenhouse et al. (1991) the neuropsychologically most impaired patients had most frequently been subject to severe angiographically proven vasospasm. This was for Stenhouse et al. (1991) the most important cause for the impairments of the patients even though a third of them also presented with hydrocephalus. Moreover, both secondary complications make it plausible that these patients must have sustained a particularly severe bleeding. Unfortunately, detailed data on the severity of the bleeding are not supplied by Stenhouse et al. (1991). In so far, the conclusion of the authors that vasospasm was the cause for the severe cognitive impairments of the patients cannot be maintained without restrictions.

Ogden, Mee and Henning (1993a) reported the results of a prospective longitudinal study according to which patients with angiographically proven vasospasm presented with a significantly worse memory performance at all follow-up appointments. In the study of Tidswell et al. (1995) new postoperative vasospasm in ACoA patients led to a poorer performance in all neuropsychological tests used, as well as to more impairments in self- and proxy-rating. A negative effect of vasospasm was seen across the entire study sample regarding performance in the WCST and impairments in daily life (Tidswell et al., 1995). Hütter and Gilsbach (1993), however, did not find any association between cognitve deficits and elevated mean blood flow velocities measured by TCD. Yet, it must be taken into account that only a loose connection exists between the mere elevation of blood flow velocities in one of the main cerebral arteries as assessed by TCD and hemodynamically relevant vasospasm. In so far, no definite conclusion about the persisting neuropsychological sequelae of vasospasm can be drawn, but it should be taken into consideration in future studies whether angiographical or doppersonographical as well as symptomatic or asymptomatic vasospasm had been present (Hütter, Kreitschmann-Andermahr and Gilsbach, 1998).

20. Prognostic factors of the neurobehavioral late result after SAH

Vilkki et al. (1990) investigated 83 patients one year after aneurysm rupture. Incomplete neurological recovery went along with impairments in verbal memory and increased cognitive inflexibility (Vilkki et al., 1990). Mercier et al. (1991) found that the neuropsychological result after discharge from hospital reliably predicted the patients, later ability to resume work. In the study by Hütter and Gilsbach (1993), a significant effect of patient age at the time of SAH emerged. At an age range of 25–67 years, older patients presented with a significantly worse concentration capacity, a poorer short-term memory and a decreased information capacity in spite of age-corrected test scores (Hütter and Gilsbach, 1993). Comparable results regarding an unfavorable prognostic effect of higher age on the neuropsychological late result after SAH were also reported by Bornstein et al. (1987). In a stepwise regression analysis with the number of cognitive deficits as factor, Hardemark et al. (1989) found that patient age at the time of SAH and the initial clinical state after Hunt and Hess were included as the exclusive predictors of later cognitive impairment.

Also according to the results of Vilkki et al. (1990), the age of patients at the time of SAH was an important predictor of social maladjustment. Mercier et al. (1991) found in 81 patients three months after aneurysm rupture that the extent of neuropsychological impairments was largely dependent on patient age and preoperative clinical state. In the study by Ogden, Mee and Henning (1993a), older patients had a significantly poorer neuropsychological result. Richardson (1991), however, was not able to find any effect of age on neuropsychological test performance of patients after aneurysm rupture in a longitudinal study. Also Tidswell et al. (1995) could not demonstrate an unfavorable effect of age in their SAH patients. Since an effect of age was found in the majority of studies, the conclusion that patient age is an important predictor of the neuropsychological late result after SAH is justified. Also regarding mortality and neurological morbidity, older patients exhibit a poorer prognosis after SAH (Lanzino et al., 1996; Gilsbach et al., 1988b).

In the study by Hütter and Gilsbach (1993) multivariate analyses showed a significantly unfavorable effect of the severity of the bleeding (Fisher CCT grading) on sensorimotor coordination (Wiener Determinationsgerät) and word fluency (FWIT). This result can be regarded as evidence for the noxious effect of subarachnoid blood especially on fronto-basal structures. Word fluency tasks exhibit a high sensitivity for the functional integrity of frontal brain structures (Hütter, 1997b). Neither vasospasm, even when rated as severe (TCD < 160 cm/sec), neurological state on admission to the unit (Hunt and Hess), interval between SAH and follow-up nor gender of the patients had a significant influence on the neuropsychological test result at follow-up (Hütter and Gilsbach, 1993). In 30 patients between seven and 42 months after aneurysm surgery, Maier-Hauff, Djouchorda and Hättig (1991) found substantial associations between the initial clinical state of the patients (Hunt and Hess) and the extent of neuropsychological impairments. However, in a study by Tidswell et al. (1995), neither the initial clinical state nor the distribution of blood on CCT exhibited an association with the cognitive deficits of the patients. Taking into account psychosocial adjustment and neuropsychological results of the patients, also Säveland et al. (1986) found that 60% patients in an initial grade I to II after Hunt and Hess had a good result. Even 70% of all patients initially grade I–II attained an overall favorable result when using a modified Fisher CCT grading. Ogden, Mee and Henning (1993a) saw a prognostically unfavorable effect of the severity of the bleeding and intracerebral or intraventricular hemorrhage with respect to cognitive capacity at the time of discharge from hospital and 12 months later. In the study by Hardemark et al. (1989) the amount of blood on initial CCT, the initial Hunt and Hess grade as well as the acute concentration of S-100 protein in CSF as an expression of the severity of the initial damage of the neurons correlated significantly with the results of a neuropsychological investigation performed two years later. Richardson (1991), however, found that the initial clinical state was not associated with neuropsychological test performance six weeks after discharge, but with cognitive capacity six months later.

When interpreting the results of the studies by Richardson (1991) and Hütter, Kreitschmann-Andermahr and Gilsbach (1998) as well as the follow-up results, it can be deduced that for the prognosis of the cognitive functional level in the acute stage of SAH the severity of the bleeding (Fisher-Score) is most relevant, but for the prediction of the persisting impairments rather the initial clinical state (Hunt and Hess) is of the greatest importance.

21. SAH as a psychological trauma

When leafing critically through the scientific literature, it becomes obvious that the frequency and severity of emotional disturbances and personality changes as a consequence of SAH are out of proportion to the, on average rather moderate, cognitive and neurological impairments of these patients (Hütter, 1998; Hütter, Kreitschmann and Gilsbach, 1995; Stegen and Freckmann, 1991; Vilkki et al., 1990; Bornstein et al., 1987; Ljunggren et al., 1985). This discrepancy can also not be explained by a psychological reaction on persisting functional deficits or the social stigma associated with "to have had trouble with the head". Therefore, the question about the possible causes for the psychological abnormalities occurring after SAH arises. A total of six hypotheses can be offered to explain this discrepancy:

1. For unknown reason, possibly already before the hemorrhage SAH patients increasingly exhibit psychological adjustment problems as compared to the normal population. However, this question can only be answered by a prospective epidemiological study;
2. The psychological abnormalities stem from brain damage that cannot be visualized by present imaging diagnostics;
3. Increased strain due to headache and a diffuse sense of impairment in combination with the feeling of a general loss of performance capacity;
4. Feelings of guilt to have caused or helped to bring about the illness or to have been punished for former misdeeds by "the scourge of God";
5. Inadequate illness coping;
6. The sudden catastrophic event of the bleeding taking place without prior warning acts as a psychological trauma leading to the symptoms of posttraumatic stress disorder (PTSD) or, below the threshold of PTSD, to posttraumatic coping difficulties (Mc Millan, 1996; American Psychiatric Association, 1994; Erikson, 1976; Horowitz, 1975).

The affected persons often experience SAH as a sudden detrimental shooting pain from the neck into the head out of any daily situation "as never before", "a crushing headache", "as struck by lightning". In an older study, Locksley (1969) came to the result that one third of the aneurysm ruptures occurred during sleep, bodily strain and under unspecific circumstances, respectively. Schievink et al. (1989) found that 43% of the aneurysm ruptures occurred in stressful situations, 34% in situations of bodily strain, i.e. lifting a heavy weight, defecation or sexual intercourse, 12% during sleep and in 11% under uncertain circumstances. Also Ogden, Mee and Henning (1993b) found a significant correlation with stressful life events and the hemorrhage in a retrospective study with 257 consecutive patients after SAH. At the time of the bleeding, 7.8% of the patients were asleep, 16.7% rested, 22.6% were moderately active and 33.5% were involved in intense activity including emotional strain and shock, while in 19.5% no activity could be identified at the time of SAH (Ogden, Mee and Henning, 1993b). In the case of spontaneous non-traumatic SAH without a proven source of the bleeding, Oder et al. (1991) described in nearly 40% of all cases a correlation between heavy bodily strain and the hemorrhage. Already Walton (1953) reported that one quarter of his patients after SAH exhibited a severe and oftentimes persisting fear of a recurrent bleeding. Logue et al. (1968) investigated 79 patients (66 operated and 13 conservatively treated) between 7 and 101 months after the acute event by a number of psychiatric tests and a psychiatric interview. Against the general expectation, the fear of a new bleeding was in 13 of the 66 operated patients (19.6%) more frequent than in patients with SAH without a proven source of the bleeding, where only one of 13 (7.6%) patient reported of such a fear. In the study of Stegen and Freckmann (1991) 79% of the patients were afraid of recurrent hemorrhage.

In order to verify the hypothesis in how far SAH can be regarded as a psychological trauma, 45 patients were investigated in an own study four years after the acute event by means of a number of questionnaires and a clinical interview (SKID) for the diagnosis of a PTSD according to DSM IV criteria (American Psychiatric Association, 1994). Moreover, for the evaluation of the extent of psychic traumatization, the German version of the Impact of Event Scale (IES) by Hütter and Fischer was used. Further questionnaires were the Beck Depression Inventory, (Beck et al., 1961), the revised version of the Freiburg Personality Inventory (FPI-R) by Fahrenberg, Hampel and Selg (1985), as well as the Aachen Life Quality Inventory (Hütter and Gilsbach, 1996b; 1995b). By means of a five-step rating (Rohrmann, 1978), the SAH patients were asked to quantify how often they were afraid of renewed hemorrhage. An extensive neuropsychological investigation had, moreover, already been performed in the acute stage of the illness. Mean age was 47 years with a range between 30 and 69 years. 20 men and 25 women after spontaneous non-traumatic SAH were in the study sample, 29 of whom had been operated upon mostly early, while no source of the bleeding had been verified in 16 patients. 80 patients who had been subject to violent crime (robbery, assault, bodily injury) 4 to 5 years ago served as the control group. In order to allow comparison to a relatively mild trauma, the IES was presented to 25 medical students who had dissected their first corpse a week before. Table 1 shows how often patients four years after SAH were still afraid of recurrent hemorrhage.

Thus, one third of the patients are frequently or even permanently afraid of recurrent hemorrhage, even four years after the acute event. A further low third still feels occasional fear of a renewed hemorrhage, so that a total of two-thirds of all patients after SAH are at least occasionally subject to anxiety about recurrent hemorrhage. It lies close at hand that fear of recurrent hemorrhage constitutes an additional psychological stress factor

Table 1. Frequency of fears about recurrent hemorrhage

Frequency	No.	%
Never	5	11
Rarely	12	27
Sometimes	13	29
Frequently	9	20
Always	6	13

next to the organic and neuropsychological impairments, that has a negative influence on the psychosocial adjustment of the affected patients.

PTSD according to DSM-IV criteria was seen in a total of 12 (26%) patients four years after SAH, 9 (31%) of whom had been operated upon and 3 (19%) who had not. Although the sample size is not large enough for statistical comparisons, as a tendency, the operated patients develop PTSD more frequently than the unoperated. In comparison to medical students after their first autopsy, the SAH patients had significantly ($p < 0.000$) higher scores in the IES subscale "Avoidance" and the IES sum score of the total amount of psychic traumatization ($p = 0.004$). On the other hand, no significant difference existed between both groups with respect to the IES subscale "Intrusion" ($p = 0.13$). As compared to victims of violence, SAH patients were significantly ($p < 0.000$) less affected by intrusions (IES subscale "Intrusion") and also exhibited a significantly ($p = 0.006$) lower extent of total psychic traumatization (IES sum score). Interestingly, no significant differences between the mean scores of the operated patients and those with SAH without a proven source of the bleeding regarding the total extent of psychic traumatization (IES sum score) or the two IES subscales "Intrusion" and "Avoidance" were found. This result is in so far surprising because the operated patients had to get over a more severe bleeding, a more severe clinical course and brain surgery. This should have had an additional traumatizing effect on the patients. On the other side, the fact that the source of hemorrhage had been excluded for all times by surgery and, therefore, on a rational basis, patients did not have to fear a recurrent bleeding, might have an unburdening effect on the operated patients. However, no significant difference with respect to fear about recurrent hemorrhage was found between the two groups ($p > 0.05$).

Among the clinical traits of the severity of illness as well as the acute course of the illness, the extent of intrusions (IES subscale "Intrusion") correlated with the initial clinical state after Hunt and Hess ($r = 0.32$; $p < 0.01$). The severity of the bleeding (Fisher Score) correlated with the frequency of intrusions ($r = 0.35; p < 0.01$) and the total severity of psychic traumatization ($r = 0.31; p < 0.01$). No substantial association emerged between the IES scores and maximal mean blood flow velocities on TCD as an indicator for the severity of vasospasm, as a potentially also psychologically incriminating complication ($p > 0.05$, respectively). The close relationship between the severity of psychic traumatization and fear of recurrent hemorrhage was verified by substantial correlations which shared approximately 40% of common variance between self-rated fear of recurrent hemorrhage and the frequency of intrusions ($r = 0.66; p < 0.001$) and the score in the IES "Avoidance" subscale ($r = 0.62; p < 0.001$) as well as the IES sum score ($r = 0.68; p < 0.001$). The IES subscale "Avoidance" correlated with $r = 0.45$ ($p < 0.001$), "Intrusion" with $r = 0.52$ ($p < 0.001$) and the IES sum score with $r = 0.51$ ($p < 0.001$) with the severity of depression (BDI). Depression, therefore, exhibited only modest associations with the severity of the psychological trauma, sharing approximately 25% of common variance. Although this points to a relationship between depression and psychic traumatization, the only moderate degree of common variance underlines the relative independence of these two constructs.

As the only neuropsychological parameter assessed four years earlier, the performance in the Go/NoGo subtest of the Zimmermann test battery (number of errors) correlated negatively with the frequency of intrusive cognitions with $r = -0.35$ ($p < 0.001$) and the IES sum score ($r = -0.25$; $p < 0.01$). No further significant correlations emerged in any of the other neuropsychological test results. Since the Go/NoGo test must be regarded as sensitive for fronto-cortical cognitive functions, this implies that impairment by intrusions increased with brain organic fronto-cortical functional impairment. Intrusions are cognitive-emotional encroachments (nightmares, mental images, compulsive thoughts) into consciousness and occur automatically or against the will of the patient. Brain organic weakening of the functional integrity of the frontal brain, therefore, leads to increased involuntary apperception of the content of a traumatic event, with the consequence of increased intrusions and, correspondingly, an intensified psychic traumatization and the associated stress reaction. According to these results this posttraumatic stress reaction can persist for several years. In the

Table 2. Correlations between the subscales of the FPI-R and the IES

FPI-R subscale	IES-Avoidance	IES-Intrusion	IES-Total score
Life-satisfaction	−0,28 ns	−0,34*	−0,33*
Ambition	−0,05 ns	−0,07 ns	−0,06 ns
Social orientation	−0,29 ns	−0,34*	−0,33*
Sensitivity	0,04 ns	0,13 ns	0,09 ns
Aggressiveness	0,25 ns	0,25 ns	0,26 ns
Strain	0,21 ns	0,35*	0,30*
Bodily complaints	0,44**	0,56**	0,55**
Bodily concern	0,23 ns	0,29 ns	0,27 ns
Social desirability	0,12 ns	0,11 ns	0,12 ns
Extraversion	−0,18 ns	−0,19 ns	−0,18 ns
Emotional lability	0,45**	0,58**	−0,55**

ns = not significant; *$p < 0{,}01$; **$p < 0{,}001$

following, Table 2 shows the correlation between the subscales of the Freiburger Personality Inventory (FPI-R) and the IES.

Mostly no or only moderate correlations emerged with the subscales of the FPI-R which hardly shared more than 10% of common variance (Table 2). This shows that psychic traumatization on the one and aspects of psychological adjustment on the other hand represent associated but independent constructs. The highest correlations were found in this respect with the extent of bodily complaints (psychosomatic disturbance) and increased emotional lability (both FPI-R) which can be assigned as symptoms to the syndrome of a PTSD. Table 3 gives an overview of the associations between the severity of psychic traumatization (IES) and self-rated impairments of quality of life (ALQI) of the patients.

The severity of traumatization correlates with increased impairments in most areas of HRQOL, which is most pronounced in the psychosocial aspect of the life quality. Remarkably, also high correlations emerged with the ALQI subscale "Cognitive capacity", which assesses day-to-day impairments of cognitive capacity. Subjective cognitive complaints as memory and concentration problems account for the core symptoms of PTSD. Even though the IES apparently assesses an independent construct of psychological strain due to a stressful event which is, however, connected to PTSD, the particularly close relationship to such symptoms which constitute a PTSD supports the validity of the IES as a measure for the evaluation of the severity of psychological traumatization extending to the scope of PTSD.

These results lead to the conclusion that spontaneous SAH independent of etiology represents a persistent psychological trauma. In up to a third of the patients, this traumatization was so severe that it led to the occurrence of PTSD. Correlation analyses show that also below the threshold of PTSD

Table 3. Correlations between the IES scores and the ALQI subscales

ALQI subscales[1]	IES-Avoidance	IES-Intrusion	IES-Total score
Activation	0,36*	0,41**	0,41**
Mobility	0,32*	0,35*	0,36*
House-work	0,22 ns	0,35*	0,30*
Social contact	0,34*	0,42**	0,40*
Family relations	0,21 ns	0,32*	0,28 ns
Free time activities	0,44**	0,54**	0,51**
Ambulation	0,23 ns	0,29 ns	0,27 ns
Communication	0,23 ns	0,28 ns	0,26 ns
Autonomy	0,08 ns	0,12 ns	0,10 ns
Cognition	0,38*	0,54**	0,49**
ALQI Total score[1]	0,44**	0,52**	0,53**
ALQI Psycho-social score	0,41**	0,49**	0,50**
ALQI Physical score	0,34*	0,39*	0,40*

ns = not significant; *p < 0,01; *p < 0,001

[1]The ALQI subscale "Work" was not included because only 19 patients worked regularly

psychological traumatization of the patients has in some areas a significant unfavorable influence on psychological adjustment (FPI-R) and health-related quality of life (ALQI), while the associations with concrete impairments in psychosocial areas of daily life are particularly pronounced (Table 2). The shared variance between depression (BDI) and the severity of psychological traumatization was at most 25%. Overall, the highest correlations emerged between the extent of psychic traumatization (IES) and those symptoms associated with PTSD. It is remarkable that frontal brain damage led to increased strain by intrusions which probably promotes increased psychological stress next to the consequences of organic brain damage. Therefore, according to these promising results, a further study with a larger number of patients as well as the inclusion of patients after accidental traumatic brain injury is called for. The traumatization of SAH patients due to the hemorrhage should, in the future, be increasingly taken into consideration for neuropsychological rehabilitation in order to prevent the occurrence of psychological disturbances and to further the later psychosocial adjustment of the affected patients in the sense of secondary prevention. The development of specific psychotherapeutic interventions tailored to patients with brain damage is a desired aim for future research in rehabilitation neuropsychology.

22. Problems of rehabilitation of patients after SAH

22.1. Spontaneous functional regeneration after SAH

According to general clinical experience, six months after aneurysm surgery functional recovery has progressed so far that this clinical state corresponds for the most part to the endpoint of clinical recovery. Essen et al. (1991) found a complex recovery curve which did not point unequivocally to the direction of functional improvement in patients after rupture and surgical repair of an intracranial aneurysm. However, also the process of functional recovery after traumatic brain injury seems to exhibit complex traits of the clinical course and, moreover, the significance of individual prognostic factors has not been elucidated fully so far (Levin, Grafman and Eisenberg, 1987). Kertesz and McCabe (1977) studied the course of functional recovery in logopedically untreated as well as treated aphasics. In the total study sample of 93 aphasics, there were also 12 patients after SAH. With respect to prognosis and functional recovery, considerable differences were found between the etiological groups. The pattern of the clinical course of aphasics due to SAH exhibited a large variability in the progression of clinical recovery. Furthermore, the clinical course was more unfavorable than in those patients with aphasia due to traumatic brain injury. The clinical course was rather comparable to that of patients with cerebral infarctions. Especially the rupture of a left-sided MCA aneurysm oftentimes led to severe and persisting aphasias according to the results of Kertesz and McCabe (1977). Artiola and Fortuny (1978) found the most pronounced improvement of cognitive deficits in patients after aneurysm rupture in the immediate postoperative phase. Afterwards, Artiola and Fortuny (1978) observed only slight improvements. McKenna et al. (1989b) investigated 83 patients in a prospective longitudinal study at discharge from hospital as well as three months and one year after the acute event by means of a neuropsychological test battery and a semi-structured interview pertaining to problems in daily life. At the time of discharge, most patients exhibited cognitive deficits, but already at follow-up three months later the cognitive level of performance had improved considerably. After one year none of the neurologically intact patients exhibited a cognitive deficit (McKenna et al., 1989b). In a further study Richardson (1991) found statistically significant improvements in spatial cognition and a vocabulary test in SAH patients.

In a case report, Hall and Young (1992) reported about a 23-years old man who suddenly developed a somnolent state with flattened affect.

A psychoorganic syndrome with auditory hallucinations and unusual associations ensued. At the neurological examination, a left-sided aneurysm of the MCA and a frontal, intracerebral bleeding, approximately 7 cm in diameter was found. Although the clinical course had been complicated, the symptoms regressed quickly postoperatively except for a residual slight aphasia and moderate memory deficits (Hall and Young, 1992). In a prospective longitudinal study, Ogden, Mee and Henning (1993a) investigated 89 patients after SAH with a mostly good neurological result at the time of discharge from hospital as well as 10 weeks and six months later. Except for tests of concentration capacity, cognitive speed and flexibility and particularly the WCST as a test relatively sensitive for frontal brain function, a considerable and significant improvement was found in all other evaluated cognitive functions. However, Ogden, Mee and Henning (1993a) did not give account on the percentage of those patients in their study sample in whom neuropsychological rehabilitation had been performed. In particular, the frequency of memory deficits between the time of discharge from the neurosurgical unit ranged from 30–88% to 8–46% at follow-up one year later depending on the function tested (Ogden, Mee and Henning, 1993a). It was, however, striking that improvements in particularly disturbed memory functions were considerably less pronounced than in initially less impaired areas of memory (Ogden, Mee and Henning, 1993a). In a prospective longitudinal study with 66 included patients, Ogden, Mee and Henning (1994) found by means of a clinical interview and a number of questionnaires 10 weeks and one year after SAH, that neither complaints about excessively increased fatigue (88.9% 10 weeks after SAH and 86.2% one year later) nor complaints about increased sensitivity to noise (54.4% 10 weeks after SAH and 55.4% one year later) had abated substantially. However, significant improvements were found regarding depressiveness (BDI), emotional adjustment and activities including social behavior within the first 12 months after SAH (Ogden, Mee and Henning, 1994). In a consecutive series of patients after aneurysm rupture, in a time span between six weeks after discharge and six months later, Richardson (1989) only saw a marginal improvement of memory performance. Also Gade (1982) reported that those patients with ruptured aneurysm of the ACoA who presented with a postoperative amnestic syndrome, did not improve in memory performance at the time of follow-up two years later. The result of Hütter and Gilsbach (1993), too, established that the temporal distance between the hemorrhage and follow-up which amounted after all to between one and four years did not exhibit any relation to neuropsychological test performance. This leads to the conclusion that at the latest one year after the hemorrhage no substantial functional regeneration takes place. The result is, however, limited by the small study sample (31 patients) and the inclusion of exclusively early operated patients who exhibited a good (GOS = I) neurological result at six-month follow-up (Hütter and Gilsbach, 1993). However, also in other studies a comparable stability of the psychological symptoms after SAH was found (Essen et al., 1991; DeSantis et al., 1989; Deruty et al., 1988; Gade, 1982).

22.2. General elements of rehabilitation after SAH

There are three levels of consequences of bodily diseases: 1. impairment as the damaged organ system, 2. disability as the impaired function and 3. handicap as the individual psychosocial consequences (World Health Organization, 1980). Rehabilitation measures should cover all three levels, with special emphasis on the levels disability and handicap. German social statutes guarantee every patient threatened by disability or incapacity to work, next to acute medical treatment, a legal claim for rehabilitation. Rehabilitation measures should be initiated as early as possible. Here, the principles "rehabilitation before retirement" and "rehabilitation before nursing" are applicable. The ultimate aim of rehabilitation must be the restitution of bodily, psychological and social integrity. Overall, social medical concepts of rehabilitation pursue the following aims (Table 1).

For the rehabilitation of patients after SAH two areas must be differentiated: 1. the overall somatic and neurological rehabilitation of bodily complaints or disturbances of function, respectively and 2. the neuropsychological rehabilitation of cognitive impairments and psychosocial problems. It is an applied principle of neuropsychological rehabilitation that at the latest after six months, according to more recent results already after 3 months after brain damage, the apex of the rehabilitation potential is already surpassed (von Cramon and Ziehl, 1989). Early rehabilitation, which is absolutely desirable, should be initiated already in the postoperative stage, if possible. Generally, the need for neuropsychological rehabilitation can be assessed on the basis of the neuropsychological investigation, but the patients' wish should also be taken into consideration. The aim of rehabilitation measures consists in the registration and facilitation of recovery tendencies of neurological and neuropsychological disturbances of function. Furthermore, compensation strategies for permanently impaired

Table 1. Aims of rehabilitation measures after SAH

1. Restauration of impaired functions
2. Optimization of residual functions
3. Acquisition of new strategies for compensation of persistent functional impairments
4. Improvement of persistence
5. Acquisition of coping strategies
6. Encouragement of illness coping
7. Information about causes and consequences of the illness
8. Acquisition of adaptive illness behavior
9. Adjustment to the affordances of work and daily life in relation to the functional capacities of the patient
10. Support of professional reintegration

functions must be trained. In patients, largely independent in daily life, the aim is to regain or ameliorate the capacity to work. The occupational and psychosocial situation of the patient must possibly be altered in so far, that the professional, familial and social handicap is diminished. Here, also social and psychological interventions are called for. In this context, outpatient rehabilitation also plays an increasing role. Since the neurological and neuropsychological impairments after SAH are, in general, not so severe, rehabilitation should be performed on an outpatient basis as far as possible. When stationary rehabilitation is unavoidable, it would be sensible to include ambulatory rehabilitation as a second step. Also the relatives play a large role in the psychosocial care of the patients.

22.3. Scientific studies on the effectiveness of neuropsychological rehabilitation measures in patients after SAH

Still in 1986, Busch was of the opinion that the prognosis of rehabilitation measures in patients after cerebrovascular diseases is worse as compared to patients with brain tumors or after traumatic brain injury (Busch, 1986). Essen et al. (1991) voiced a comparable scepticism. Busch later reported on the neuropsychological deficits and the success of rehabilitation in 171 patients after SAH due to aneurysm rupture who had been referred to stationary rehabilitation (Busch, 1987). An aphasic language disturbance was found in 24% of the patients, cognitive deficits in 79% and a psychoorganic syndrome in 38%. Certainly, these figures are not representative for the entire collective of survivors after the rupture of an intracranial aneurysm, but constitute a selected sample based on the indication for rehabilitation, which should have led to an increased part of neurologically/neuropsychologically impaired patients. Busch (1987) determined that in 36% of the patients an improvement of an aphasic language disturbance, in 49% an increase of the cognitive capacity and in 36% a restitution of a psychoorganic syndrome could be achieved during a seven weeks long rehabilitation, but only in 11% a restitution of the capacity for work. This result, however, constitutes a twofold discrepancy, for once with the only moderate degree of cognitive impairments of SAH patients, and second, with the considerable improvements of cognitive functions as a consequence of rehabilitation as reported by Busch (1987). This implies that in SAH patients rehabilitation measures influence individual cognitive functions positively, but the goal of thorough psychosocial and occupational reintegration is not achieved. On the other hand, Hampl et al. (1990) found that 47% of the SAH patients began to work after the end of rehabilitation, while 48% of the patients began to work again without rehabilitation. However, the patients without rehabilitation were considerably more impaired. This result by Hampl et al. (1990) points to an at least gradual effect of rehabilitation also in SAH patients. Here, the so far overlooked (also in the planning of rehabilitation measures) aspect of the psychological traumatization of the patients must be mentioned.

A pharmacological treatment concept for the cognitive impairments of patients after SAH was evaluated by Maier-Hauff (1991). Maier-Hauff (1991) conducted a placebo-controlled double blind study on the efficacy of an gingko-biloba extract (LI 1370) on the mental capacity of 50 patients 7–42 months after aneurysm surgery. After 12 weeks of therapy, significant positive effects on verbal short-term memory and the number of errors in the Go/NoGo test were found (Maier-Hauff, 1991). Säveland et al. (1988) found in a study on the cognitive impairments of 56 patients after SAH and early surgery, that two years later no difference existed between the 21 patients who had received nimodipine intravenously in the acute stage and those not treated with nimodipine. Vilkki et al. (1989) also saw no differences in neuropsychological test performance between 27 patients treated with nimodipine and 29 patients who had received a placebo.

In contrast to purely somatic therapies whose effectiveness can be measured in terms of the incidence of treatment-induced neurological disturbances, remission and survival rates, evaluation of the success of rehabilitation is much more difficult. Next to the symptom-related assessment of the success of neuropsychological rehabilitation in the sense of the diminution or resolution of cognitive deficits, in the future also the HRQOL should be recruited as an assessment criterion, as already postulated by Busch (1986). The ultimate goal of all rehabilitation efforts should not consist in the amelioration of isolated functional deficits but in the integration of the patient into everyday life and the amelioration of impairments in daily life.

23. Closing discussion and outlook

Due to the introduction of the operating microscope, modern aneurysm clips, the concept of early surgery and a more refined intensive care management, the prognosis of patients with ruptured intracranial aneurysms has improved substantially. Nevertheless, neuropsychological studies show a marked discrepancy between a good neurological result according to the Glasgow Outcome Scale (GOS = I) and the cognitive and psychosocial functional level of the patients surviving SAH. Surprisingly, no differences between the impairments of operated patients and those having sustained spontaneous non-traumatic SAH without a proven source of the bleeding could be demonstrated.

Already the first scientific accounts of the sequelae of ruptured intracranial aneurysms contain some descriptions of the psychological symptoms accompanying the clinical picture. Therefore, scientific interest in the investigation of the neuropsychological consequences of this illness and the clarification of its causes exists for quite some time. However, neuropsychological research was focused before all on ruptured aneurysms of the ACoA. This is probably best explained by the fact that with this aneurysm location, frequently severe psychopathological and neuropsychological abnormalities as i.e. amnestic syndromes up to Korsakoff psychosis have been observed. However, due to methodological weaknesses of older studies, neither the relative incidence of Korsakoff syndrome after rupture and surgical repair of aneurysms of the ACoA is proven conclusively, nor can a greater incidence of this symptomatology in comparison to other aneurysm locations be assumed unequivocally. Since the older studies are based before all on small study samples or selected individual cases, for a long time the hypothesis had been adopted that ACoA aneurysm location is closely associated with amnestic syndromes. In the literature on this topic, some authors compounded a threefold association between ACoA aneurysm location, frontal brain damage and the presence of anterograde amnesia. However, no single one of the postulated relations can be maintained. Neither did ACoA aneurysm location lead particularly often to frontal brain damage nor to an amnestic syndrome, nor is frontal brain damage the prerequisite for the occurrence of memory deficits (including anterograde amnesia or Korsakoff syndrome) in patients after aneurysm rupture.

The critical analysis of the scientific literature reveals, however, that the earlier macrosurgical techniques used during the surgical repair of a ruptured aneurysm of the ACoA played a decisive role in the occurrence of an amnestic syndrome. It can be postulated that a lacking specific effect of

ACoA aneurysm location can be traced back to an improvement of surgical techniques which make it meanwhile possible to spare the small perforators originating from the ACoA. Moreover, for a long time – before all in older studies on the neuropsychological sequelae of ruptured aneurysms of the ACoA – the hypothesis has been advanced that specific consequences of the rupture of intracranial aneurysms in dependence of location existed. On the other hand, next to an increasing number of studies by other research groups, also the own results with the comparison of consecutive series of patients with ruptured intracranial aneurysms of different locations reveal no specific effect of aneurysm location. This also holds true for the rupture of aneurysms of the ACoA whose neuropsychological sequelae differ neither quantitatively nor qualitatively from those of other aneurysm locations. In own studies, no general unfavorable effect of the surgical repair of a ruptured intracranial aneurysm could be found. When analyzing the neuropsychological sequelae of different surgical measures and events, it became evident that the duration of temporary clipping of vessels can lead to an additional impairment of the patients in the short as well as in the long run, even if the exact conditions for such an unfavorable effect of temporary clipping are, at present, still unclear. This should be elucidated in future studies.

Even if there is at present still a lack of empirical studies on the neuropsychological sequelae of other aneurysm locations than the ACoA, there is some evidence that particularly severe neuropsychological impairments occur after the rupture of aneurysms of the basilar circulation. The results of our own studies demonstrating that also spontaneous non-traumatic SAH without a proven source of the bleeding leads to a comparable pattern of neurobehavioral impairments as SAH due to aneurysm rupture speak against specific effects of aneurysm location. On the basis of these results, in the present work the hypothesis is formulated and supported with data of empirical studies that the neuropsychological sequelae of SAH are independent of aneurysm location, but rather depend on the anatomical pattern of the bleeding and herewith associated secondary complications such as disturbances of CSF circulation and vasospasm. The results of our own studies support this hypothesis and show that SAH leads to frontally accentuated brain damage which results of the anatomy of the initial hemorrhage. This frontal morphological damage can oftentimes not be made visible by imaging diagnostics such as CCT or MRI but is reflected in neuropsychological tests sensitive for frontal brain function. Also the impairments in daily life and the emotional changes of SAH patients can at least partially be put down to latent frontal brain damage.

However, there exists a disparity in patients after SAH between functional and emotional impairments as well as impairments in daily life. In order to explain this discrepancy, in the present work the hypothesis is advanced that patients after SAH are traumatized psychologically due to the hemorrhage. It was demonstrated in one study that even four years after the bleeding one third of the operated patients suffered of post-traumatic stress disorder (PTSD) according to DSM-IV criteria. Moreover, important associations between the extent of psychological traumatization and impairments in daily life, in particular, and, to a lesser extent, emotional disturbances were found.

Between 30–50% of all patients after SAH showed persisting cognitive deficits and disturbances of emotional adjustment. Neuropsychological tests covering functions of attention and short-term memory appear to be especially sensitive for the assessment of the late sequelae after SAH. For this reason such tests should be contained in all test batteries by means of which patients after SAH are investigated. A practical consequence of the relevant investigations on the neuropsychological sequelae of SAH is that the true extent of the illness and treatment sequelae can only be evaluated by the use of a differentiated neuropsychological test battery that goes beyond the measurement of general intelligence. A patient who has survived SAH without neurological deficits still has a high probability to exhibit neuropsychological deficits. Therefore, early neuropsychological diagnostics and herewith associated well-timed onset of neuropsychological rehabilitation as well as early information and counseling for patients and relatives are of particular importance in order to prevent the occurrence of secondary psychosocial adjustment disturbances.

References

Aaronson NK (1988) Quality of life: What is it? How should it be measured? Oncology 2: 69–74

Aaslid R, Markwalder TM, Nornes H (1982) Noninvasive transcranial Doppler ultrasound recording of flow velocities in basal cerebral arteries. J Neurosurg 57: 769–774

Adams JE, Witt JA (1964) The use of the otological microscope in the surgery of aneurysms. Paper presented at the 17th Annual Meeting of the Neurological Society of America. Litchfield Park, Arizona

Adams HP, Kassell NF, Torner JC, Sahs AL (1983) CT and clinical correlations in recent aneurysmal subarachnoid hemorrhage: a preliminary report of the Cooperative Aneurysm Study. Neurology 33: 981–988

Adams JP, Kassell NF, Torner JC (1985) Usefulness of computed tomography in predicting outcome after aneurysmal subarachnoid hemorrhage: a preliminary report of the Cooperative Aneurysm Study. Neurology 35: 1263–1267

Adams HP, Kassell NF, Torner JC, Haley EC (1987) Predicting cerebral ischemia after aneurysmal subarachnoid hemorrhage: influences of clinical condition, CT results, and antifibrinolytic therapy. A report of the Cooperative Aneurysm Study. Neurology 37: 1586–1591

Albright F (1929) The syndrome produced by aneurysm at or near the function of the internal carotid artery and the circle of Willis. Johns Hopkins Hosp Bull 44: 215–245

Alexander MSM, Dias PS, Uttley D (1986) Spontaneous subarachnoid hemorrhage and negative cerebral panangiography. J Neurosurg 64: 537–542

Alexander MP, Freedman M (1984) Amnesia after anterior communicating artery aneurysm rupture. Neurology 34: 752–757

Allison RS, Hurwitz LJC (1967) On perseveration in aphasics. Brain 90: 429–448

Amelang M, Borkenau P (1982) Über die faktorielle Struktur und externe Validität einiger Fragebogen-Skalen zur Erfassung von Dimensionen der Extraversion und emotionalen Labilität. Z Diff Diagnost Psychol 3: 119–145

American Psychiatric Association (1994) Diagnostic and statistical manual of mental disorders, fourth edition. Washington DC: American Psychiatric Association

Amthauer R (1953) Der Intelligenz-Struktur-Test IST. Göttingen: Hogrefe Verlag

Anderson C, Laubscher S, Burns R (1996) Validation of the short form 36 (SF-36) health survey questionnaire among strong patients. Cerebrovasc Dis 6: S7

Anderson SW, Tranel D, Damasio H (1988) The use of tumor and stroke patients in neuropsychological research: a methodological critique. J Clin Exp Neuropsychol 10: S32

Anderson SW, Damasio H, Jones RD, Tranel T (1991) Wisconsin Card Sorting Test performance as a measure of frontal lobe damage. J Clin Exp Neuropsychol 13: 909–922

Anzai Y, Simon HA (1979) The theory of learning by doing. Psychol Rev 86: 124–140

Arena R, Gainotti G (1978) Constructional apraxia and visuopractic disabilities in relation to laterality of cerebral lesions. Cortex 14: 463–473

Arnold U, Pössl J (1995) Psychopathologische Diagnostik. In: von Cramon DY, Mai N, Ziegler W (Hrsg) Neuropsychologische Diagnostik. London, Weinheim: Chapman & Hall, pp 287–310

Artiola I, Fortuny L (1978) Improvement in visual and haptic deficits in a neurosurgical population. Dissertation abstracts international 38: 6214 B

Artiola I, Fortuny L, Prieto-Valiente L (1981) Long-term prognosis in surgically treated intracranial aneurysm. Part 2: Morbidity. J Neurosurg 54: 55–43

Ask-Upmark E, Ingvar D (1950) A follow-up examination of 138 cases of subarachnoid haemorrhage. Acta Med Scand 88: 15–31

Aboderin I, Venables G (1996) For the Pan European Consensus Meeting on Stroke Management in Europe. J Int Med 240: 173–180

Attenberry-Bennett J, Barth JT, Loyd B, Lawrence EC (1989) The relationship between behavioural and cognitive deficits, demographics and depression in patients with minor head injuries. Clin Neuropsychol 5: 114–117

Auer S, Gallhofer B, Auer LM (1985) What does full recovery after acute aneurysm operation mean? A psychological study. In: Auer LM (ed) Timing of aneurysm surgery. Berlin, New York: Walter de Gruyter, pp 129–132

Auer LM, Schneider GH, Auer T (1986) Computerized tomography and prognosis in early aneurysm surgery. J Neurosurg 65: 217–221

Awad IA, Carter P, Spetzler RF, Medina M, Williams FW (1987) Clinical vasospasm after subarachnoid hemorrhage: response to hypervolemic hemodilution and arterial hypertension. Stroke 18: 365–372

Bailes JE, Spetzler RF, Hadley MN, Baldwin HZ, Zabramski JM (1990) Management morbidity and mortality of poor-grade aneurysm patients. J Neurosurg 72: 559–566

Bak JS, Greene RL (1981) A review of the performance of aged adults on various Wechsler Memory Scale subtests. J Clin Psychol 37: 186–188

Bamford J, Sandercock P, Dennis M, Burn J, Warlow C (1990) A prospective study of acute cerebrovascular disease in the community: the Oxfordshire Community Stroke Project-1981–86. J Neurol Neurosurg Psychiat 53: 16–22

Barbarotto R, De Santis A, Basso A, Spagnoli D, Capitani E (1989) Neuropsychological follow-up of patients operated for aneurysms of the middle cerebral artery and posterior communicating artery. Cortex 25: 275–288

Barker FG, Ogilvy CS (1996) Efficacy of prophylactic nimodipine for delayed ischemic deficit after subarachnoid hemorrhage: A metaanalysis. J Neurosurg 84: 405–414

Batjer H, Samson D (1986) Intraoperative aneurysm rupture: incidence, outcome and suggestions for surgical management. Neurosurgery 18: 701–707

Bäumler G (1985) Der Farbe-Wort-Interferenztest (FWIT). Göttingen: Hogrefe Verlag

Beadles CF (1907) Aneurisms of the larger cerebral arteries. Brain 30: 285–336

Beck AT, Ward CH, Mendelson M, Mock J, Erbaugh J (1961) An inventory for measuring depression. Arch Gen Psychiat 4: 561–571

Benton AL (1968) Differential effects of frontal lobe disease. Neuropsychologia 6: 53–60

Benton AL (1981) Der Benton Test. Bern, Stuttgart, Wien: Huber Verlag

Ben-Yishay Y, Piasetsky EB, Rattok J (1987) A systematic method for ameliorating disorders in basic attention. In: Meier MJ, Benton AL, Diller L (eds) Neuropsychological rehabilitation. Edinburgh, London: Churchill Livingstone, pp 165–181

Bergner M, Bobbitt RA, Carter WB, Gilson BS (1981) The Sickness Impact Profile: Development and final revision of a health status measure. Med Care 19: 787–805

Bertalanffy H, Seeger W (1991) The dorsolateral, suboccipital, transcondylar approach to the lower clivus and anterior portion of the craniocervical junction. Neurosurgery 29: 815–821

Beukelman DR, Flowers, CF, Swanson PD (1980) Cerebral disconnection associated with anterior communicating artery aneurysm: Implications for evaluation of symptoms. Arch Phys Med Rehabil 61: 18–23

Blumer D. Benson DG (1975) Personality changes with frontal and temporal lobe lesions. In: Benson DF, Blumer D (eds) Psychiatric aspects of neurologic disease. New York: Grune & Stratton, pp 151–169

Bonita R, Thompson S (1985) Subarachnoid hemorrhage: epidemiology, diagnosis, management and outcome. Stroke 16: 591–594

Borkenau P, Amelang M (1986) Zur faktorenanalytischen Kontrolle sozialer Erwünschtheitstendenzen. Eine Untersuchung anhand des Freiburger Persönlichkeits-Inventars. Zeitschr Diff Diagnost Psychol 7: 17–28

Bornstein RA, Weir BK, Petruk KC, Disney LB (1987) Neuropsychological function in patients after subarachnoid hemorrhage. Neurosurgery 21: 651–654

Botterell EH, Lougheed WM, Scott JW, Vandewater SL (1956) Hypothermia and interruption of carotid, or carotid and vertebral circulation, in the surgical management of intracranial aneurysms. J Neurosurg 13: 1–42

Bramwell B (1886) Clinical and pathological memoranda. IV. Case of aneurism of the right internal artery. Edinburgh Med J 32: 97–101

Brandt L, Sonesson B, Ljunggren B, Säveland H (1987) Ruptured middle cerebral artery aneurysm with intracerebral hemorrhage in younger patients appearing moribund: emergency operation? Neurosurgery 20: 925–929

Brickenkamp R (1978) Test d2 Aufmerksamkeits-Belastungs-Test. Göttingen: Hogrefe Verlag

Brinker T, Seifert V, Dietz H (1992) Cerebral blood flow and intracranial pressure during experimental subarachnoid haemorrhage. Acta Neurochir 115: 47–52

Brion S, Derome P, Guiot G, Teitgen M (1968) Syndrome de Korsakoff par aneurisme de l'artere communicante anterieure; le probleme des syndromes de Korsakoff par hemorrhagie meningee. Rev Neurol 118: 293–299

Brismar J, Sundbärg G (1985) Subarachnoid hemorrhage of unknown origin: prognosis and prognostic factors. J Neurosurg 63: 349–354

Broadbent DN (1958) Perception and communication. London: Pergamon Press

Brouwers PJAM, Dippel DWJ, Vermeulen M, Lindsay KW, Hasan D, van Gijn J (1993) Amount of blood on computed tomography as an independent predictor after aneurysm rupture. Stroke 24: 809–814

Bullinger M, Ludwig M, von Steinbüchel N (1991) Lebensqualität bei kardiovaskulären Erkrankungen. Göttingen, Toronto, Zürich: Hogrefe Verlag

Bullinger M (1997) Gesundheitsbezogene Lebensqualität und subjektive Gesundheit. Psychother Psychosom Med Psychol 47: 76–91

Busch G (1986) Rehabilitation bei malignen Hirntumoren. Neurochirurgia 25: 35–38

Busch G (1987) Rehabilitation of patients with organic brain damage after diseases requiring neurosurgery. In: Wüllenweber R, Klinger M, Brock M (eds) Advances in Neurosurgery. Vol 75. Berlin, Heidelberg, New York: Springer, pp 255–258

Canavan AGM, Janota I, Schurr PH (1985) Luria's frontal lobe syndrome: psychological and anatomical considerations. J Neurol Neurosurg Psychiat 48: 1049–1053

Carter BS, Buckley D, Ferrano R, Manno E, Ogilvy CS (1996) Long term outcome after subarachnoid hemorrhage: physical, psychiatric, and social recovery in Hunt & Hess Grade I–III patients. J Neurosurg 84: 355A–356A

Chansky N (1967) Validity of the Benton Visual Retention Test. Percept Mot Skills 24: 1126

Charbel FT, Ausman JI, Dias FG, Malik GM, Dujovny M, Sanders J (1991) Temporary clipping in aneurysm surgery: Technique and results. Surg Neurol 36: 83–90

Chyatte D, Fode NC, Sundt TM (1988) Early versus late intracranial aneurysm surgery in subarachnoid hemorrhage. J Neurosurg 69: 326–331

Chyatte D, Chen TL, Bronstein K, Brass LM (1994) Seasonal fluctuation in the incidence of intracranial aneurysm rupture and its relationship to changing climatic conditions. J Neurosurg 81: 525–530

Chelune GJ, Heaton RK, Lehman AW (1986) Neuropsychological and personality correlates of patients complaints of disability. In: Goldstein G, Tarter RE (eds) Advances in clinical neuropsychology Vol III. New York, London: Plenum Press, pp 95–126

Chernik DA, Tucker M, Gigli B, Yoo K, Paul K, Laine H, Siegel JC (1992) Validity and reliability of the Neurobehavioral Assessment Scale. J Clin Psychopharmacol 12: 43–48

Cioffi F, Pasqualin A, Cavazzani P, Da Pian R (1989) Subarachnoid haemorrhage of unknown origin: clinical and tomographical aspects. Acta Neurochir 97: 31–39

Compton JS, Redmond S, Symon L (1987) Cerebral blood velocity in subarachnoid haemorrhage: A transcranial Doppler study. J Neurol Neurosurg Psychiat 50: 1499–1503

Corkin S, Cohen NJ, Sullivan EV, Clegg RA, Roden TJ (1985) Analyses of global memory impairments of different etiologies. Ann New York Acad Sci 444: 10–40

Crockett D, Bilsker D, Hurwitz T, Kozak J (1986) Clinical utility of three measures of frontal lobe dysfunction in neuropsychiatric samples. Intern J Neurosci 30: 241–248

Crowell RM, Morawetz RB (1977) The anterior communicating artery has significant branches. Stroke 8: 272–273

Cubbitt AW (1930) Spontaneous subarachnoid hemorrhage with Korsakoff's psychosis. Br Med J 9: 212–213

Dahl G (1972) WIP-Revidierter Wechsler Intelligenztest. Meisenheim: Hain Verlag

Dam H, Peterson HE, Ahlgren P (1989) Depression among patients with stroke. Acta Psychiat Scand 80: 118–124

Damasio AR, Graff-Radford NR, Eslinger PJ, Damasio H, Kassell N (1985a) Amnesia following basal forebrain lesions. Arch Neurol 43: 263–271

Damasio AR, Eslinger PJ, Damasio H, Graff-Redford NR (1985b) Multimodal amnesic syndrome following bilateral temporal and basal forebrain damage. Arch Neurol 42: 252–259

Damasio AR, Tranel D, Damasio H (1989) Amnesia caused by herpes simplex encephalitis, infarctions of the basal forebrain, Alzheimer's disease and anoxia/ischemia. In: Squire L, Gainotti G (eds) Handbook of neuropsychology Vol 3. Amsterdam: Elsevier, pp 149–166

Dandy WE (1938) Intracranial aneurysm of the internal carotid artery, cured by operation. Ann Surg 107: 654–657

Dandy WE (1939) The treatment of internal carotid aneurysms within the cavernous sinus and cranial chamber. Report of 3 cases. Ann Surg 109: 689–711

Dandy WE (1944) Intracranial arterial aneurysms. Ithaca, New York: Comstock, Cornell University, pp 1–147

David M, Pertuiset B, Guyot JF (1968) La cure radicale des aneurysmes de la communicante anterieure sans resection cerebrale chez le malade conscient. Considerations cliniques postoperatoire. Rev Neurol 118: 150–151

DeLuca J (1990) Predicting behavioral patterns following anterior communicating artery aneurysm. Arch Phys Med Rehabil 71: 828

DeLuca J, Cicerone KD (1991) Confabulation following aneurysm of the anterior communicating artery. Cortex 27: 417–423

DeLuca J (1992a) Rehabilitation of confabulation: The issue of unawareness of deficit. Neuro Rehabil 2: 23–30

DeLuca J (1992b) Cognitive dysfunction after aneurysm of the anterior communicating artery. J Clin Exp Neuropsychol 14: 924–934

DeLuca J (1993) Predicting neurobehavioral patterns following anterior communicating artery aneurysm. Cortex 29: 639–647

Deruty R, Patet JD, Mottolese C, Portilla F (1988) Long-term outcome of the management of ruptured intracranial aneurysm: Review of 328 consecutive patients treated over a period of 12 years. Neurol Res 10: 217–220

Deruty R, Pelissou-Guyotat I, Mottolese C, Bognar L, Oubouklik A (1992) Surgical management of unruptured intracranial aneurysms. Acta Neurochir 119: 35–41

Deruty R, Pelissou-Guyotat I, Mottolese C, Amat D, Bognar L (1995) Level of consciousness and age as prognostic factors in aneurysmal SAH. Acta Neurochir 132: 1–8

De Santis A, Laiacona M, Barbarotto R, Basso A, Villani R, Spagnoli D, Capitani E (1989) Neuropsychological outcome of patients operated upon for an intracranial aneurysm.

Analysis of general prognostic factors and of the effects of the location of the aneurysm. J Neurol Neurosurg Psychiat 52: 1123–1140
Devinsky O, Morrell MJ, Vogt BA (1995) Contributions of anterior cingulate cortex to behavior. Brain 118: 279–306
Disney L, Weir B, Grace M (1988) Factors influencing the outcome of aneurysm rupture in poor grade patients: A prospective series. Neurosurgery 23: 1–9
Dorman P, Farrell B, Dennis M, Sandercock P (1996) Health related quality of life after stroke: a randomized comparison of the EuroQuol and SF-36 questionnaires in 2252 survivors of acute stroke. Cerebrovasc Dis 6: S152
Dott NM (1933) Intracranial aneurysms: cerebral arterio-graphy: surgical treatment. Edinburgh Med J 40: 219–240
Dott NM (1969) Intracranial aneurysmal formations. Clin Neurosurg 16: 1–16
Drake CG, Vanderlinden RG (1967) The late consequences of incomplete surgical treatment of cerebral aneurysms. J Neurosurg 27: 226–238
Drake CG (1979) Giant intracranial aneurysms: experience with surgical treatment in 174 patients. Clin Neurosurg 26: 12–95
Drake CG (1981) Progress in cerebrovascular disease. Management of cerebral aneurysm. Stroke 12: 273–283
Drake CG, Freedman AH, Peerless SJ (1984) Failed aneurysm surgery – reoperation in 115 cases. J Neurosurg 61: 848–856
Drewe EA (1974) The effect of type and area of brain lesion on Wisconsin Card Sorting Test performance. Cortex 10: 159–170
Drewe EA (1975) Go-no go learning after frontal lobe lesions in humans. Cortex 11: 8–16
Ebrahim S, Barer D, Nouri F (1986) Use of the Nottingham Health Profile with patients after stroke. J Epidemiol Comm Health 40: 166–169
Ecker A, Riemenschneider PA (1951) Arteriographic demonstration of spasm of the intracranial arteries with special reference to saccular arterial aneurysms. J Neurosurg 8: 660–667
Ellenbogen RG, Scott RM (1991) Transfalcine approach to a callosomarginal artery aneurysm. Neurosurgery 29: 140–143
Erikson KT (1976) Loss of communality at Buffalo Creek. Am J Psychiatry 133: 302–305
Erikson RC, Scott ML (1977) Clinical memory testing: A review. Psychol Bull 84: 1130–1149
Eskesen V, Soerensen EB, Rosenoern J, Schmidt K (1984) The prognosis in subarachnoid hemorrhage of unknown etiology. J Neurosurg 61: 1029–1031
Essen CV, Jakobson K-E, Löfgren J, Roos A, Starmark J-E, Stephensen H, Bitting M, Svensson E (1991) Complexity of recovery following ruptured intracranial aneurysm and operation. Paper presented at the Annual Congregation of the Sweedish Medical Association in Stockholm, Sweden
Fahrenberg J, Hampel R, Selg H (1984) Das Freiburger Persönlichkeitsinventar FPI. Revidierte Fassung FPI-R. Göttingen: Hogrefe Verlag
Fahrenberg J, Hampel R, Selg H (1985) Die revidierte Form des Freiburger Persönlichkeitsinventars FPI-R. Diagnostica 31: 1–21
Feinstein AR, Josephy BR, Wells CK (1986) Scientific and clinical problems in index of functional disability. Ann Intern Med 105: 413–420
Ferbert A, Hubo I, Biniek R (1992) Non-traumatic subarachnoid hemorrhage with normal angiogram. J Neurol Sci 107: 14–18
Feuerberg I, Lindquist C, Lindquist M, Steiner L (1987) Natural history of postoperative aneurysm rests. J Neurosurg 66: 30–34
Fields F (1971) Relative effects of brain damage on the Wechsler memory and intelligence quotients. Dis Nerv Syst 32: 673–675
Findlay JM, Weir BKA, Kanamaru K, Grace M, Baughman R (1990) The effect of timing of intrathecal fibrinolytic therapy on cerebral vasospasm in a primate model of subarachnoid hemorrhage. Neurosurgery 26: 201–206

Findlay JM, Weir BKA, Kassell NF, Disney LB, Grace MGA (1991) Intracisternal recombinant tissue plasminogen activator after aneurysmal subarachnoid hemorrhage. J Neurosurg 75: 181–188

Findlay JM, Grace MGA, Weir BKA (1993) Treatment of intraventricular hemorrhage with tissue plasminogen activator. Neurosurgery 32: 941–947

Fisher CM, Roberson GH, Ojemann RG (1977) Cerebral vasospasm with ruptured saccular aneurysm – the clinical manifestations. Neurosurgery 1: 245–258

Fisher CM, Kistler JP, Davis JM (1980) Relation of cerebral vasospasm to subarachnoid hemorrhage visualized by computerized tomographic scanning. Neurosurgery 6: 1–9

Flanagan JC (1975) The concept of quality of life for American community members. Soc Ind 63: 56–59

Flanagan JC (1982) Measurement of quality of life: current state of the art. Arch Phys Med Rehabil 63: 56–59

Flateau E (1921) Sur les hemorrhagies meningees idiopathique. Gaz des Hopitaeux 94: 1077–1081

Forssell A, Larsson C, R'nnberg J, Fodstad H (1995) CT assessment of subarachnoid haemorrhage. A comparison between different CT methods of grading subarachnoid haemorrhage. Br J Neurosurg 9: 21–27

Fox JL (1983) Intracranial aneurysms. Vol I–III. New York, Berlin: Springer

Friedman WA, Chadwick GM, Verhoeven FJS, Mahla M, Day AL (1991) Monitoring of somatosensory evoked potentials during surgery for middle cerebral artery aneurysms. Neurosurgery 29: 83–88

Fuster JM (1989) The prefrontal cortex, 2nd ed. New York: Raven Press

Gade A (1982) Amnesia after operations on aneurysms of the anterior communicating artery. Surg Neurol 18: 46–49

Gade A, Mortensen EL (1990) Temporal gradient in the remote memory impairment of amnesic patients with lesions in the basal forebrain. Neuropsychologia 28: 985–1001

Gallhofer B, Auer LM (1982) Spontaneous course after subarachnoid haemorrhage: Evaluation of 109 patients. Acta Neurochir 63: 67–70

Gerber CJ, Lang DA, Neil-Dwyer G, Smith PW (1993) A simple scoring system for accurate prediction of outcome within four days of a subarachnoid haemorrhage. Acta Neurochir 122: 11–22

Gilsbach JM, Eggert HR (1983) Early operations on ruptured aneurysms. In: Jensen HP, Brock M, Klinger M (eds) Advances in Neurosurgery Vol 2. Berlin, Heidelberg, New York: Springer, pp 79–82

Gilsbach JM, Harders AG, Eggert HR, Hornyak ME (1988a) Early aneurysm surgery: a 7 year clinical practice report. Acta Neurochir 90: 91–102

Gilsbach JM, Harders AG, Hornyak ME, Seeger W (1988b) Is early aneurysm surgery indicated in the elderly? Geriat Cardiovasc Med 1: 73–79

Gilsbach JM (1988) Nimodipine in the prevention of ischemic deficits after aneurysmal subarachnoid hemorrhage – an analysis of recent clinical studies. Acta Neurochir 95: 41–50

Gilsbach JM, Harders AG (1989) Morbidity and mortality after early aneurysm surgery–a prospective study with nimodipine prevention. Acta Neurochir 96: 1–7

Gilsbach JM, Reulen HJ, Ljunggren B, Brandt L, von Holst H, Mokry M, van Essen C, Conzen MA (1990) Early aneurysm surgery and preventive therapy with intravenously administered nimodipine: a multicenter, double-blind, dose-comparison study. Neurosurgery 26: 458–464

Gilsbach JM, Poeck K, Piscol K (1993) Hirngefäßaneurysmen. In: Hopf HC, Poeck K, Schliack H (Hrsg) Neurologie in Klinik und Praxis. Vol III. Stuttgart, New York: Thieme, 2.1–2.25

Gilsbach JM, Mayfrank L, Lennartz B (1996) Versorgung des Schädel-Hirn-Traumas im neurochirurgischen Zentrum. Chirurg 67: 1114–1122

Goldberg E, Costa LD (1986) Qualitative indices in neuropsychological assessment. An extension of Luria's approach to executive deficit following prefrontal lesions. In: Grant I, Adams K (eds) Neuropsychological assessment of neuropsychiatric disorders. New York: Oxford University Press, pp 68–84

Goldberg E, Bilder RM (1987) The frontal lobes and hierarchical organisation of cognitive control. In: Perecman E (ed) The frontal lobes revisited. New York: IRBN Press, pp 159–187

Goldenberg G, Wimmer A, Holzner F, Wessely P (1985) Apraxia of the left limbs in a case of callosal disconnection: The contribution of medial frontal lobe damage. Cortex 21: 135–148

Goldflam S (1923) Beitrag zur Ätiologie und Symptomatologie der Spontanen Subarachnoidalen Blutungen. Deutsch Z Nervenh 76: 158–182

Gomez FB, Dujovny M, Umansky F, Berman SK, Diaz FG, Ausman J, Mirchandani HG, Ray WJ (1986) Microanatomy of the anterior cerebral artery. Surg Neurol 26: 129–141

Grady CL, Grimes AM, Petronas N (1989) Divided attention as measured by dichotic speed performance in dementia of the Alzheimer type. Arch Neurol 46: 317–330

Graf CJ (1971) Prognosis for patients with non-surgically treated aneurysms. J Neurosurg 35: 438–443

Greenberg IM (1984) Cerebral aneurysm rupture during neurosurgery. Neurosurgery 15: 243–245

Gronwall D, Wrightson P (1974) Delayed recovery of intellectual function after minor head injury. Lancet 2: 995–997

Grote E, Hassler W (1988) The first critical minutes after subarachnoid hemorrhage. Neurosurgery 22: 654–661

Guglielmi G, Vinuela F, Sepetka I, Macellari V (1991) Electrothrombosis of saccular aneurysms via endovascular approach. Part 1: Electrochemical basis, technique, and experimental results. J Neurosurg 75: 1–7

Guillard A, Fenelon G, Mahieux F (1991) Les alterations cognitives au cours de la maladie de parkinson. Rev Neurol 147: 337–355

Gurusinghe NT, Richardson AE (1984) The value of computed tomography in aneurysmal subarachnoid hemorrhage. The concept of CT-score. J Neurosurg 60: 763–770

Hahlweg K, Kühnlein I (1981) Die Bewährung des Benton Test in der psychiatrischen Klinik: I Aufgabenanalyse und Bestimmung der inneren Konsistenz; II Konstruktvalidität und differentielle Gültigkeit. Diagnostica 27: 1–17

Hall AJ (1929) Three cases of spontaneous subarachnoid hemorrhage: With especial reference to the occurrence of massive albuminuria and Korsakow's syndrome. Br Med J 8: 1025–1028

Hall DP, Young SA (1992) Frontal lobe cerebral aneurysm rupture presenting as psychosis. J Neurosurg 55: 1207–1208

Hall JC, Toal R (1957) Reliability (internal consistency) of the Wechsler Memory Scale. J Consult Psychol 21: 131–135

Hall S, Bornstein RA (1991) The relationship between intelligence and memory following mi nor head injury: greater impairment in memory than in intelligence. J Neurosurg 75: 378–381

Halstead WC (1947) Brain and intelligence: a quantitative study of the frontal lobes. Chicago: University Press of Chicago

Hamburger C, Schönberger J, Lange M (1992) Management and prognosis of intracranial giant aneurysms. A report on 58 cases. Neurosurg Rev 15: 97–103

Hampl J, Berger H, Degenhard M, Irle E, Kunert J, Kunze S (1990) Postoperative long-term results after aneurysm surgery among patients treated with Nimodipine. In: Bushe KA, Brock M, Klinger M (eds) Advances in neurosurgery. Vol 18. Berlin, Heidelberg, New York: Springer, pp 227–232

Handa Y, Hayashi M, Takeuchi H, Kubota T, Kobayashi H, Kawano H (1992) Time course of the impairment of cerebral autoregulation during chronic cerebral vasospasm after subarachnoid hemorrhage in primates. J Neurosurg 76: 493–501

Harders AG, Gilsbach JM (1987) Time course of blood velocity changes related to vasospasm in the circle of Willis measured by transcranial Doppler ultrasound. J Neurosurg 66: 718–728

Harders AG, Laborde G, Droste DW (1992) Mental activity and changes in cerebral blood flow evaluated by transcranial Doppler sonography. In: Schmiedek P, Einhäupl K, Kirsch CN (eds) Stimulated cerebral blood flow. Berlin, Heidelberg, New York: Springer, pp 200–211

Hardemark HG, Almquist O, Johansson T, Pahlman S, Persson L (1989) S-100 protein in cerebrospinal fluid after aneurysmal subarachnoidal haemorrhage: relation to functional outcome, late CT, and SPECT changes, and signs of higher cortical dysfunction. Acta Neurochir 99: 135–144

Hasan D, Tanghe HLJ (1992) Distribution of cisternal blood in patients with acute hydrocephalus after subarachnoid hemorrhage. Ann Neurol 31: 374–378

Hasan D, Van Peski J, Loeve I, Krenning EP, Vermeulen M (1992) Single photon emission computed tomography in patients with acute hydrocephalus or with cerebral ischemia after subarachnoid haemorrhage. J Neurol Neurosurg Psychiat 54: 490–493

Hashimoto N, Handa H (1982) The fate of untreated symptomatic cerebral aneurysms: Analysis of 26 patients with clinical course of more than five years. Surg Neurol 18: 21–26

Hassler O (1961) Morphological studies on the large cerebral arteries with reference to the aetiology of subarachnoid hemorrhage. Arch Neurol Scand (Suppl) 159: 1–14

Hauerberg J, Eskesen V, Rosenorn J (1994) The prognostic value of intracerebral haematoma as shown on CT scanning after aneurysmal subarachnoid haemorrhage. Br J Neurosurg 8: 333–339

Hautzinger M (1981) Kognitive Therapie der Depression. München, Wien, Baltimore: Urban und Schwarzenberg

Heaton RK, Pendleton MG (1981) Use of neuropsychological tests to predict adult patients everyday functioning. J Consult Clin Psychol 49: 807–821

Heaton RK, Chelune GJ, Talley JL, Kay GG, Curtiss G (1993) Wisconsin Card Sorting Test manual 2nd ed. Odessa, Florida: Psychological Assessment Resources

Hecaen H, Albert ML (1975) Disorders of mental functioning related to frontal lobe pathology. In: Benson DF, Blumer D (eds) Psychiatric aspects of neurologic diseases. New York: Grune & Stratton, pp 137–147

Heiskanen O, Vilkki J (1981) Intracranial arterial aneurysm in children and adolescents. Acta Neurochir 59: 55–63

Heiskanen O, Poranen A, Kuurne T, Valtonen S, Kaste M (1988) Acute surgery for intracerebral haematomas by rupture of an intracranial arterial aneurysm. A prospective randomized study. Acta Neurochir 90: 81–83

Herman E (1925) Quelques considerations sur les hemorrhagies sous-arachnoidiennes. Rev Neurol 1: 993–996

Hernesniemi JM, Vapalathi M, Niskanen M, Tapaninaho A, Kari A, Luukkonen M, Puranen M, Saari T, Pajpar M (1993) One-year outcome in early aneurysm surgery: a 14 years experience. Acta Neurochir 122: 1–10

Hijdra A, Brouwers PJ, Vermeulen M, van Gijn J (1990) Grading the amount of blood on computed tomograms after subarachnoid hemorrhage. Stroke 21: 1156–1161

Hodes JE, Aymard A, Gobin YP, Rüfenacht D, Bien S, Reizine D, Gaston A, Merland JJ (1991) Endovascular occlusion of intracranial vessels for curative treatment of unclippable aneurysms. J Neurosurg 75: 694–701

Hodgson J (1815) A treatise on the diseases of arteries and veins, containing the pathology and treatment of aneurysms and wounded arteries. London, pp 76–78

Holms JM (1958) The medical management of subarachnoid haemorrhage. Br Med J 1: 788–790

Hori S, Suzuki J (1979) Early intracranial operations for ruptured aneurysms. Acta Neurochir 46: 93–104

Horn W (1983) Das Leistungsprüfsystem LPS. Göttingen: Hogrefe Verlag

Hornyak M, Gilsbach JM, Harders A (1991) Clinical significance of computed tomography in early aneurysm surgery. Neurochirurgia 34: 135–140

Horowitz M (1975) Intrusive and repetitive thoughts after experimental stress. Arch Gen Psychiatry 32: 1457–1463

Hounsfield GN (1973) Computerized transverse axial scanning (tomography). Br J Radiol 46: 1016–1047

House A, Dennis M, Warlowe C, Hawton K, Molyneux A (1990) Mood disorders after stroke and their relation to lesion location – A CT scan study. Brain 113: 1113–1129

Huber M, Emunds H, Herholz K, Karbe H, Heiss WD (1990) Prognostische Bedeutung des regionalen zerebralen Glukosestoffwechsels bei zerebralem Insult. In: von Wild K, Janzik HH (Hrsg) Neurologische Frührehabilitation. München, Bern, Wien, San Francisco: Zuckschwerdt Verlag, pp 153–171

Huber W, Poeck K, Weniger D, Willmes K (1983) Aachener Aphasie Test. Göttingen: Hogrefe Verlag

Hughes JT, Oppenheimer DR (1969) Superficial siderosis of the central nervous system. Acta Neuropathol 13: 56–74

Hughes JT, Schianchi PM (1978) Cerebral artery spasm: a histological study of necropsy of the blood vessels in cases of subarachnoid hemorrhage. J Neurosurg 48: 515–525

Hunt WE, Meagher JN, Barnes JE (1960). The management of intracranial aneurysm. J Neurosurg 19: 34–40

Hunt WE, Hess RM (1968) Surgical risk as related to time of intervention in the repair of intracranial aneurysms. J Neurosurg 28: 14–20

Hutchinson TA, Boyd NF, Feinstein AR, Gonda A, Hollomby D, Vrowat B (1979) Scientific problems in clinical scales as demonstrated in the Karnofsky index of performance status. J Chron Dis 32: 661–663

Hussein S, Archilli MM (1996) Microanatomy and supplying areas of the anterior cerebral artery-anterior communicating artery-complex (ACA-ACoA-complex). Zbl Neurochir 57: S25

Hütter BO (1990) Anforderungen an die Untersuchung der Lebensqualität von Patienten mit Hirntumoren. 5. Tagung der Neuroonkologischen Arbeitsgruppe der Deutschen Gesellschaft für Neurochirurgie in Köln. Book of Abstracts, pp 17–18

Hütter BO, Gilsbach JM (1992) Cognitive deficits after rupture and early repair of anterior communicating artery aneurysms. Acta Neurochir 116: 6–13

Hütter BO, Gilsbach JM (1993) Which neuropsychological deficits are hidden behind a good outcome (Glasgow = I) after aneurysmal subarachnoid hemorrhage? Neurosurgery 33: 999–1006

Hütter BO, Gilsbach JM, Kreitschmann I (1994) Is there a difference in cognitive deficits after aneurysmal subarachnoid hemorrhage and subarachnoid hemorrhage of unknown origin? Acta Neurochir 127: 129–135

Hütter BO, Gilsbach JM (1995a) Introspective capacities in patients after subarachnoid hemorrhage. J Clin Exp Neuropsychol 17: 499–517

Hütter BO, Gilsbach JM (1995b) Lebensqualität bei Patienten mit Hirnschädigung: Entwicklung und psychometrische Überprüfung des Aachener Lebensqualitätsinventars. In: Schwarz R, Bernhard J, Flechtner H, Küchler Th, Hürny Ch (Hrsg) Lebensqualität in der Onkologie. Vol II. München, Bern, Wien, New York: Zuckschwerdt Verlag, pp 132–138

Hütter BO, Gilsbach JM, Kreitschmann I (1995) Quality of life and cognitive deficits in patients after subarachnoid haemorrhage. Br J Neurosurg 9: 465–475

Hütter BO, Engell B, Huber W (1995) Entwicklung eines Instrumentariums zur Erfassung der Lebensqualität bei Aphasikern. Nervenheilkunde 14: 34–37

Hütter BO, Gilsbach JM (1996a) Early neuropsychological sequelae of aneurysm surgery and subarachnoid haemorrhage. Acta Neurochir 138: 1370–1379

Hütter BO, Gilsbach JM (1996b) Das Aachener Lebensqualitätsinventar für Patienten mit Hirnschädigung: Entwicklung und methodische Gütekriterien. In: Möllers HJ, Engel RR, Hoff P (Hrsg) Befunderhebung in der Psychiatrie: Lebensqualität, Negativsymptomatik und andere aktuelle Entwicklungen. Wien, Berlin, New York: Springer, pp 83–101

Hütter BO, Claßen K, Gilsbach JM (1996) Kognition und Lebensqualität von Patienten mit frontalen, umschriebenen niedriggradigen Gliomen. Zbl Neurochir 57: S63–64

Hütter BO, Würtemberger G (1997a) Validity and Reliability of the German version of the Sickness Impact Profile in patients with chronic obstructive pulmonary disease. Psychology and Health 12: 149–159

Hütter BO, Würtemberger G (1997b) Lebensqualität bei chronisch-obstruktiven Lungenerkrankungen: Psychometrische Gütekriterien der deutschen Version des Sickness Impact Profiles (SIP) und erste Ergebnisse der Anwendung. Pneumologie 51: 108–114

Hütter BO (1997a) Neuropsychologische Folgen von Frontalhirnschädigungen I: Funktionelle Neuroanatomie und kognitive Beeinträchtigungen. Nervenheilkunde 16: 317–322

Hütter BO (1997b) Neuropsychologische Folgen von Frontalhirnschädigungen II: Kritische Überlegungen zum sogenannten "Frontalhirnsyndrom", Fragen der Diagnostik und Theorien der Frontalhirnfunktion. Nervenheilkunde 16: 429–434

Hütter BO, Niemann K, Coenen VA, Gilsbach JM (1997a) Disorders of memory functions and the hippocampal formation: Findings in patients with well-defined unilateral lesions. Exp Brain Res 117: S38

Hütter BO, Niemann K, Coenen VA, Küker W, Gilsbach JM, Thron A (1997b) Digital 3-D lesion analysis of the hippocampal formation: Neuropsychological effects of well-defined unilateral lesions. In: Hütter BO, Gilsbach JM (eds) Neuropsychology in neurosurgery, psychiatry and neurology. Aachen: Augustinus Verlag, pp 35–36

Hütter BO (1998) Psychologic adjustment in patients after subarachnoid hemorrhage. Neuropsychiat Neuropsychol Behav Neurol 11: 22–30

Hütter BO, Kreitschmann-Andermahr I, Gilsbach JM (1998) Cognitive deficits in the acute stage after subarachnoid hemorrhage. Neurosurgery 43: 1054–1065

Hütter BO, Kreitschmann-Andermahr I, Mayfrank L, Spetzger U, Rohde V, Gilsbach JM (1999) Functional outcome after aneurysmal subarachnoid hemorrhage. Acta Neurochir 72: 157–174

Hütter BO, Fischer G (2000) Clinimetric evaluation of the German version of the Impact of Event Scale (IES). J Traum Stress (in press)

Hütter BO, Mayfrank L, Gilsbach JM (submitted) Neuropsychological sequelae of lumbar puncture and shunting in patients with malresorptive hydrocephalus after subarachnoid hemorrhage: report of four cases.

Ichise M, Chung DG, Wang P, Wortzman G, Gray BG, Franks, W (1994) Technetium-99-HMPAO Spect CT and MRI in the evaluation of patients with chronic traumatic brain injury: A correlation with neuropsychological performance. J Nucl Med 35: 217–226

Inagawa T, Yamamoto M, Kamiya K (1990) Effect of clot removal on cerebral vasospasm. J Neurosurg 72: 224–230

Inagawa T, Kamiya K, Matsuda (1991) Effect of continuous cisternal drainage on cerebral vasospasm. Acta Neurochir 112: 28–36

Inagawa T (1994) Timing of admission and management outcome in patients with subarachnoid hemorrhage. Surg Neurol 41: 268–276

Irle E, Wowra B, Kunert HJ, Hampl J, Kunze S (1992a) Memory disturbance following anterior communicating artery rupture. Ann Neurol 31: 473–480

Irle E, Wowra B, Kunert J, Peper M, Hampl J, Kunze S (1992b) Differential disturbances of memory and mood following striatum and basal forebrain lesions in patients with ruptures of the anterior communicating artery. In: Piscol M, Klinger M, Brock M (eds) Advances in neurosurgery, Vol 20. Berlin, Heidelberg, New York: Springer, pp 191–197

Jabre A, Symon L (1987) Temporary vascular occlusion during aneurysm surgery. Surg Neurol 27: 47–63

Jane JA, Kassell NF, Torner JC, Winn HR (1985) The natural history of aneuryms and arteriovenous malformations. J Neurosurg 62: 321–323

Jennett B, Bond M (1967) Assessment of outcome after severe brain damage. A practical scale. Lancet 1: 480–484

Jennett B, Teasdale G (1977) Aspects of coma after severe head injury. Lancet 23: 878–881

Jennett B, Snoek J, Bond MR, Brooks W (1981) Disability after severe head injury: observations on the use of the Glasgow Outcome Scale. J Neurol Neurosurg Psychiat 44: 285–293

Johnson RJ, Potter JM, Reid RG (1958) Arterial spasm in subarachnoid haemorrhage. J Neurol Neurosurg Psychiat 21: 58

Juul R, Fredriksen TA, Ringkjoeb R (1986) Prognosis in subarachnoid hemorrhage of unknown etiology: mechanical considerations. J Neurosurg 64: 359–362

Kahnemann D (1973) Attention and effort. Englewood Cliffs, NJ: Prentice Hall

Kaku Y, Yonekawa Y, Tsukahara T, Kazekawa K (1992) Superselective intra-arterial infusion of papaverine for the treatment of cerebral vasospasm after subarachnoid hemorrhage. J Neurosurg 77: 842–847

Kapur N, Coughlan AK (1980) Confabulation and frontal lobe dysfunction. J Neurol Neurosurg Psychiat 43: 461–463

Karnath O, Zimmermann P, Wallesch CW (1991) Mental planning and anticipatory processes with acute and chronic frontal lobe lesions: A comparison of maze performance in routine and non-routine situations. Neuropsychologia 29: 271–290

Karnofsky DA, Burchenal JH (1949) The clinical evaluation of chemotherapeutic agents in cancer. In: McCleod CM (ed) Evaluation of chemotherapeutic agents. New York: Columbia University Press, pp 191–205

Kassell NF, Boarini DJ, Adams HP, Sahs AL, Graf CJ, Torner HC, Gerk MK (1981) Overall management of ruptured aneurysm: comparison of early and late operation. Neurosurgery 9: 120–128

Kassell NF, Torner JC (1983) Aneurysmal rebleeding: a preliminary report from the Cooperative Aneurysm Study. Neurosurgery 13: 479–481

Kassell NF, Sasaki T, Colohan AR, Nazar G (1985) Cerebral vasospasm following aneurysmal subarachnoid hemorrhage. Stroke 16: 562–572

Kassell NF, Torner JC, Haley EC, Jane JA, Adams HP, Kongable GL, and participants (1990a) The international cooperative study on the timing of aneurysm surgery. Part I: Overall management results. J Neurosurg 73: 18–36

Kassell NF, Torner JC, Jane JA, Haley EC, Adams HP and participants (1990b) The international cooperative study on the timing of aneurysm surgery. Part II: Surgical results. J Neurosurg 73: 37–47

Keen WW (1890) Intracranial lesions. Med News NY 57: 443

Kertesz A, McCabe P (1977) Recovery patterns and prognosis in aphasia. Brain 100: 1–18

Kessler RC, Price RH, Wortmann CB (1985) Social factors in psychopathology: stress, social support and coping processes. Ann Rev Psychol 53: 531–572

Kidooka M, Nakasu Y, Watanabe K, Matsuda M, Handa J (1987) Monitoring of somatosensory evoked potentials during aneurysm surgery. Surg Neurol 27: 69–76

Kim ChJ, Cervos-Navarro J, Pätzold C, Tokuriki Y, Tabeke Y, Hori K (1992) In vivo study of flow pattern at human carotid bifurcation with regard to aneurysm development. Acta Neurochir 115: 112–117

Klebelsberg D (1960) Das Wiener Determinationsgerät. Diagnostica 6: 165–166

Koeleveld RF, Heilman CB, Kluczink RP, Shucart WA (1991) De novo development of an aneurysm: case report. Neurosurgery 29: 756–759

Klonoff PS, Snow WG, Costa LD (1986) Quality of life in patients 2 to 4 years after closed head injury. Neurosurgery 19: 735–743

Koenig GH, Marshall WH, Poole GJ, Kramer RA (1979) Rupture of intracranial aneurysms during cerebral angiography: report of ten cases and review of the literature. Neurosurgery 5: 314–324

Krampen G (1986) Zur Validität der deutschen Form des 16 PF: Faktorielle Validität und Beziehungen zum FPI. Diagnostica 32: 91–99

Kraus JF (1987) Epidemiology of head injury. In: Cooper PR (ed) Head injury, 2nd ed. Baltimore: Williams and Wilkins, pp 1–19

Kreitschmann I, Hütter BO, Gilsbach JM (1995) Katecholamin-induzierte Hypertension bei schweren prolongierten Vasospasmen nach SAB-klinische Ergebnisse und Lebensqualität. In: Jerusalem F, Reis F (Hrsg) Verhandlungen der Deutschen Gesellschaft für Neurologie. Bonn: Kilun Verlag, pp 416–418

Kreitschmann-Andermahr I, Hütter BO, Gilsbach JM (1996) Lebensqualität und neurologisches Ergebnis nach Behandlung schwerer prolongierter Vasospasmen nach SAB mittels induzierter Hypertension. In: Böker DK (Hrsg) Neue Aspekte zu Pathogenese und Therapie des zerebralen Vasospasmus. Zülpich: Biermann Verlag, pp 148–151

Kreitschmann-Andermahr I, Gilsbach JM (1996) Prävention und Therapie des Vasospasmus. In: Böker DK (Hrsg) Neue Aspekte zu Pathogenese und Therapie des zerebralen Vasospasmus. Zülpich: Biermann Verlag, pp 74–86

Laiacona M, De Santis A, Barbarotto R, Basso A, Spanioli D, Capitani E (1989) Neuropsychological follow-up of patients operated for aneursyms of the anterior communicating artery. Cortex 25: 261–273

Lanzino G, Kassell NF, Germanson TP, Kongable GL, Truskowski LL, Torner JC, Jane JA, and the participants (1996) Age and outcome after aneurysmal subarachnoid hemorrhage: why do older patients fare worse? J Neurosurg 85: 410–418

Larsson C, Rönnberg J, Forssell A, Nilsson LG, Lindberg M, Ängquist KA (1989) Verbal memory function after subarachnoid haemorrhage determined by the localisation of the ruptured aneurysm. Br J Neurosurg 3: 549–560

Lebert H (1866) Über die Aneurysmen der Hirnarterien. Eine Abhandlung in Briefen an Herrn Geheimrat Prof. Dr. Frerichs. Berl Klin Wochenschr 20: 209–212; 22: 229–231; 24: 249–251; 28: 281–285; 34: 336–338; 35: 345–347; 40: 386–390; 42: 402–405

Leng NRC, Parkin AJ (1988) Double dissociation of frontal dysfunction in organic amnesia. Br J Clin Psychol 27: 359–362

LeRoux PD, Haglund MM, Newell DW, Grady SM, Winn HR (1992) Intraven tricular hemorrhage in blunt head trauma: an analysis of 43 cases. Neurosurgery 31: 678–685

LeRoux PD, Elliott JP, Newell DW, Grady MS, Winn HR (1996a) The incidence of surgical complications is similar in good and poor grade patients undergoing repair of ruptured anterior circulation aneurysms: a retrospective review of 355 patients. Neurosurgery 38: 887–895

LeRoux PD, Elliott JP, Newell DW, Grady MS, Winn HR (1996b) Predicting outcome in poor-grade patients with subarachnoid hemorrhage: a retrospective review of 159 aggressively managed cases. J Neurosurg 85: 39–49

Levin HS, Grafmann J, Eisenberg HM (1987) Neurobehavioral recovery from head injury. New York, Oxford: Oxford University Press

Levin HS, Goldstein FC, Ghostine SY, Weiner RL, Crofford MJ, Eisenberg HM (1987) Hemispheric disconnection syndrome persisting after anterior cerebral artery aneurysm rupture. Neurosurgery 6: 831–838

Lezak MD (1982) The problem of assessing executive functions. Int J Psychol 17: 81–97

Lezak MD (1983) Neuropsychological assessment, 2nd ed. New York, Oxford: Oxford University Press

Lipper S, Morgan D, Krigman R, Staab EV (1978) Congenital saccular aneurysm in a 19-day old neonate: case report and review of the literature. Surg Neurol 10: 161–165

Lindquist G, Norlen G (1966) Korsakoff's syndrome after operation on ruptured aneurysm of the anterior communicating artery. Acta Neurol Scand 42: 24–34

Lindquist G (1975) Lesions due to aneurysms. 7th International Congress of Neuropathology. Hungary: Budapest 1–7 Sept. 1974. Excerpta Medica, pp 209–210

Linn FHH, Rinkel GJE, Algra A, van Gijn J (1996) Incidence of subarachnoid hemorrhage. Stroke 27: 625–629

Ljunggren B, Säveland H, Brandt L, Kagström E, Rehncrona S, Nilsson PE (1983) Temporary clipping during early operation for ruptured aneurysm: preliminary report. Neurosurgery 12: 525–530

Ljunggren B, Sonesson B, Säveland H, Brandt L (1985) Cognitive impairment and adjustment in patients without neurological deficits after aneurysmal SAH and early operation. J Neurosurg 62: 673–679

Ljunggren B, Brandt L, Säveland H, Sonesson B, Romner B, Zygmont S, Andersson KE, Mellegard P, Ryman T (1987) Management of ruptured intracranial aneurysm: A review. Br J Neurosurg 1: 9–32

Ljunggren B, Fodstad H, van Essen C, Säveland H, Brandt L, Hillmann J, Romner B, Algers G (1988) Aneurysmal subarachnoid haemorrhage: overall outcome and incidence of early recurrent haemorrhage despite a policy of acute stage operation. Br J Neurosurg 2: 49–53

Ljunggren B, Sharma S, Buchfelder M (1993) Intracranial aneurysms. Neurosurg Quarterly 3: 120–152

Locksley HB (1969) Natural history of subarachnoid hemorrhage, intracranial aneurysms, and arteriovenous malformations: based on 6368 cases in the cooperative study. II. In: Sahs AL, Perret GE, Locksley HB, Nishioka H (eds) Intracranial aneurysms and subarachnoid hemorrhage. Philadelphia: JB Lippincott, pp 58–108

Logue V, Durward M, Pratt RTC, Piercy M, Nixon WLB (1968) The quality of survival after rupture of an anterior cerebral aneurysm. Br J Psychiat 114: 137–160

Lunsford LD, Maroon JC, Vega A (1977) Amnestic syndrome in limbic lesions. Report of three cases. Surgical Forum 28: 481–484

Luria AR (1969) Frontal lobe syndroms. In: Vinken P, Bruyn G (eds) Handbook of clinical neurology, Vol 2. Localisation in clinical neurology. Amsterdam: North Holland, pp 725–757

Luria AR (1973) The working brain. New York: Basic Books

Luria AR (1976) The neuropsychology of memory. Washington: Winston & Sons, pp 34–52

Magnus V (1927) Aneurysm of the internal carotid artery. JAMA 88: 1712–1713

Mahoney FI, Barthel DW (1965) Functional evaluation: The Barthel index. Md State Med J 14: 61–65

Maier-Hauff K, Djoucharda D, Hättig H (1991) Die Bedeutung neuropsychologischer Untersuchungen für die Beurteilung nach SAB und Aneurysmaoperation. In: Kongressband der II. Arbeitstagung der Deutschen Gesellschaft für Rehabilitation, pp 29–32

Maier-Hauff K (1991) LI 1370 nach zerebraler Aneurysma-Operation: Wirksamkeit bei ambulanten Patienten mit Störungen der Hirnleistungsfähigkeit. Münch Med Wochenschr 133: S34–S37

Marchel A, Bidzinski J, Bojarski P (1991) formation of new aneurysms. Report of 5 cases. Acta Neurochir 112: 96–99

Marinkovic S, Milisavljevic M, Marinkovic Z (1990) Branches of the anterior communicating artery. Acta Neurochir 106: 78–85

Markowitsch HJ (1984) Can amnesia be caused by damage of a single brain structure? Cortex 20: 27–45

Matsumara A, Meguro K, Tsurushima H, Kikuchi Y, Wada M, Nakata Y (1990) Magnetic resonance imaging of spinal cord injury without radiologic abnormality. Surg Neurol 33: 281–283

Matsuda M, Shiino A, Handa J (1990) Sequential changes of cerebral blood flow after aneurysmal subarachnoid haemorrhage. Acta Neurochir 105: 98–106

Maurice-Williams RS, Willison JR, Hatfield R (1991) The cognitive and psychological sequelae of uncomplicated aneurysm surgery. J Neurol Neurosurg Psychiat 54: 335–340

Mayfrank L, Lippitz B, Groth M, Bertalanffy H, Gilsbach JM (1993) Effect of recombinant tissue plasminogen activator on clot lysis and ventricular dilatation in the treatment of severe intraventricular hemorrhage. Acta Neurochir 122: 32–38

Mayfrank L (1997) Pathophysiologie und Behandlung von Ventrikelblutungen Erwachsener: Experimentelle und klinische Untersuchungen. Unveröffentlichte Habilitationsschrift, Medizinische Fakultät der RWTH Aachen

Mayfrank L, Delsing P, Kissler J, Raoofi R, Weis J, Küker W, Gilsbach JM (1997a) The effects of tissue-type plasminogen activator (tPA) on clot lysis and ventricular dilation in a new experimental model of intraventricular hemorrhage. In: Böker DK (ed) Therapeutic concepts in spontaneous intracerebral hemorrhage. Zülpich: Biermann Verlag, pp 31–35

Mayfrank L, Kissler J, Raoofi R, Delsing P, Weis J, Küker W, Gilsbach JM (1997b) Ventricular dilatation in experimental intraventricular hemorrhage. Characterization of CSF dynamics and the effects of fibrinolytic treatment. Stroke 28: 141–148

McCormick WF, Rosenfield DB (1973) Massive brain hemorrhage. A review of 144 cases and an examination of their causes. Stroke 4: 946–954

McCormick WF (1985) Pathology of closed head injury. In: Wilkins R, Rengachery S (eds) Neurosurgery Vol 1. New York: McGraw-Hill, pp 1544–1569

McGlynn SM, Shacter DL (1989) Unawareness of deficits in neuropsychological syndromes. J Clin Exp Neuropsychol 11: 143–205

McKenna P, Willison JR, Lowe D, Neil-Dwyer G (1989a) Cognitive outcome and quality of life one year after subarachnoid hemorrhage. Neurosurgery 24: 361–367

McKenna P, Willison JR, Lowe D, Neil-Dwyer G (1989b) Recovery after subarachnoidal haemorrhage. Br Med 299: 485–487

McKissock W, Paine KWE, Walshe LS (1960) An analysis of the results of treatment of ruptured intracranial aneurysms. Report on 722 consecutive cases. J Neurosurg 17: 762–776

McMillan TM (1996) Post-traumatic stress disorder following minor and severe closed head injury: 10 single cases. Brain Injury 10: 749–758

McSweeny AJ, Grant I, Heaton RK, Prigatano GP, Adams KM (1985) Relationship of neuropsychological status to everyday functioning in healthy and chronically ill persons. J Clin Exp Neuropsychol 7: 281–291

Menon D, Weir B, Overton T (1981) Ventricular size and cerebral blood flow following subarachnoid hemorrhage. J Comput Assist Tomogr 5: 328–333

Mercier P, Le Gall D, Aubin G, Joseph PA, Alhayek G, Guy G (1991) Interet du bilan neuropsychologique dans les aneurysmes arteriels cerebraux operes. Neurochirurgie 37: 32–39

Mesulam MM (1985) Patterns in behavioral neuroanatomy: association areas, the limbic system, and hemispheric specialisation. In: Mesulam MM (ed) Principles of behavioral neurology. Philadelphia: FA Davis Company, pp 2–70

Mesulam MM (1986) Frontal cortex and behavior. Ann Neurol 19: 320–325

Mesulam MM (1990) Large scale neurocognitive networks and distributed processing for attention, language and memory. Ann Neurol 28: 597–613

Milhorat TH, Krautheim M (1986) Results of early and delayed operations for ruptured intracranial aneurysms in two series of 100 consecutive patients. Surg Neurol 26: 123–128

Milner B (1963) Effects of different brain lesions on cardsorting. Arch Neurol 9: 90–100

Milner B (1965) Visually-guided maze learning in man: effects of bilateral hippocampal, bilateral frontal-lobe lesions and unilateral cerebral lesions. Neuropsychologia 3: 317–338

Mizukami M, Kawase T, Usami T, Tazawa T (1982) Prevention of vasospasm by early operation with removal of subarachnoid blood. Neurosurgery 10: 301–307

Mohr G, Ferguson G, Khan M, Malloy D, Watts R, Benoit B, Weir B (1983) Intraventricular hemorrhage from ruptured aneurysm. J Neurosurg 58: 482–487

Momma F, Wang AD, Symon L (1987) Effects of temporary arterial occlusions on somatosensory evoked response in aneurysm surgery. Surg Neurol 27: 343–352

Moniz E (1927) L'encephalographie arterielle, son importance dans la localisation des tumeurs cerebrales. Rev Neurol 2: 72–90

Mooig JJ, Buchthal A, Belopavlovic M (1987) Somatosensory evoked potential monitoring of temporary middle cerebral artery occlusion during aneurysm operation. Neurosurgery 21: 492–496

Morecraft RJ, Geula C, Mesulam MM (1992) Cytoarchitecture and neural afferents of orbitofrontal cortex in the brain of the monkey. J Comp Neurol 323: 341–358

Morecraft RJ, Geula C, Mesulam MM (1993) Architecture of connectivity within a cingulo-fronto-parietal neurocognitive network for directed attention. Arch Neurol 50: 279–284

Mountz JM, McGillicuddy JE, Wilson MW, Bartold SP, Siegal EM (1991) Pre- and post-operative cerebral blood flow changes in subarachnoid haemorrhage. Acta Neurochir 109: 30–33

Mourier KL, Gelbert F, Assouline E, Mouret C, Reizine D, Raggueneau JL, George B (1991) MRI in multiple vascular lesions: identification of the ruptured malformation. Acta Neurochir 112: 83–87

Nattrass FJ (1928) Aneurysm of the carotid artery in the cavernous sinus: ligature of the internal carotid: recovery. Edinburgh Med J 35: 30–32

Nebes RD, Brady CB (1989) Focused and divided attention in Alzheimer's disease. Cortex 25: 305–315

Nelson RJ, Roberts J, Rubin C, Walker V, Ackery DM, Pickard JD (1991) Association of hypovolemia after subarachnoid hemorrhage with computed tomographic scan evidence of raised intracranial pressure. Neurosurgery 29: 178–182

Nestor PG, Parasuraman R, Haxby JV (1991) Divided attention and metabolic brain dysfunction in mild dementia of the Alzheimer's type. Neuropsychologia 29: 379–387

Nibbelink DW, Torner JC, Henderson W (1977) Intracranial aneurysms and subarachnoid hemorrhage – report on a randomized treatment study. A regulated bed rest. Stroke 8: 202–218

Nishioka H, Torner JC, Graf CJ, Kassell NF, Sahs AL, Goettler LL (1984) Cooperative study of intracranial aneurysm and subarachnoid haemorrhage: a long prognostic study. III. Subarachnoid haemorrhage of undetermined aetiology. Arch Neurol 41: 1147–1151

Niskanen MM, Hernesniemi JA, Vapalathi MP, Kari A (1993) One-year outcome in early aneurysm surgery: prediction of outcome. Acta Neurochir 123: 25–32

Norlen G, Olivecrona H (1953) The treatment of aneurysms of the circle of Willis. J Neurosurg 10: 404–415

Norlen G, Lindquist G (1964) The anatomy of memory. Lancet i: 335

Norlen G (1965) Some aspects of the surgical treatment of intracranial aneurysms. Neurol Med Chir (Tokyo) 7: 14–27

Norlen G (1975) Experiences with intracranial aneurysm surgery: results in early operations. Caracas: Apartado de Actas y Trabajos del XVI Congreso Latino-Americano de Neurochirurgia, pp 235–245

Nornes H (1973) The role of intracranial pressure in the arrest of hemorrhage in patients with ruptured intracranial aneurysm. J Neurosurg 39: 220–234

Nornes H (1978) Cerebral arterial flow dynamics during aneurysm haemorrhage. Acta Neurochir 41: 39–48

Nowak G, Schwachenwald R, Arnold H (1994) Early management in poor grade aneurysm patients. Acta Neurochir 126: 33–37

Nyström SHM (1973) Psychodynamics in subarachnoid hemorrhage. A study based on 1183 patients. Helsinki: TA Sahalan Kirjapaino

Oder W, Kollegger H, Zeiler K, Dal-Bianco P, Wessely P, Deecke L (1991) Subarachnoid hemorrhage of unknown etiology: early prognostic factors for long-term functional capacity. J Neurosurg 74: 601–605

O'Donnell WE, DeSoto CB, Reynolds D (1984a) Sensitivity and specificity of the Neuropsychological Impairment Scale. J Clin Psychol 40: 553–557

O'Donnell WE, Reynolds D, DeSoto CB (1984b) Validity and reliability of the Neuropsychological Impairment Scale. J Clin Psychol 40: 549–553

Ogawa A, Sato H, Sakurai Y, Yoshimoto T (1991) Limitation of temporary vascular occlusing during aneurysm surgery. Surg Neurol 36: 453–457

Ogden JA, Levin PL, Mee EW (1990) Long-term neuropsychological and psychosocial effects of subarachnoid hemorrhage. Neuropsychiat Neuropsychol Behav Neurol 3: 260–274

Ogden JA, Mee EW, Henning M (1993a) A prospective study of impairment of cognition and memory and recovery after subarachnoid hemorrhage. Neurosurgery 33: 572–587

Ogden JA, Mee EW, Henning M (1993b) Life-events stress: a significant precursor to subarachnoid hemorrhage. Neuropsychiat Neuropsychol Behav Neurol 6: 219–228

Ogden JA, Mee EW, Henning M (1994) A prospective study of psychosocial adaptation following subarachnoid haemorrhage. Neuropsychol Rehabil 4: 7–30

Ogden JA, Utley T, Mee EW (1997) Neurological and psychosocial outcome 4 to 7 years after subarachnoid hemorrhage. Neurosurgery 41: 25–34

Ogilvy CS, Poletti CE (1991) Clipping of an aneurysm 20 years after encasement with methylacrylate. J Neurosurg 75: 305–307

Öhman J, Heiskanen O (1988) Effect of nimodipine on the outcome of patients after aneurysmal subarachnoid hemorrhage and surgery. J Neurosurg 69: 683–686

Öhman J, Servo A, Heiskanen O (1991a) Long-term effects of nimodipine on cerebral infarcts and outcome after aneurysmal subarachnoid hemorrhage and surgery. J Neurosurg 74: 8–13

Öhman J, Servo A, Heiskanen O (1991b) Risk factors for cerebral infarction in good-grade patients after aneurysmal subarachnoid hemorrhage and surgery: a prospective study. J Neurosurg 74: 14–20

Okawa K, Maeda S, Nukui H, Kawafuchi J (1980) Psychiatric symptoms in ruptured anterior communicating artery aneurysms: Social prognosis. Acta Psychiat Scand 61: 306–312

Orgass B (1982) Deutsche Bearbeitung des Token Tests von E DeRenzi und LA Vignolo. Weinheim: Beltz Verlag

Origitano TC, Wascher TM, Reichman OH, Anderson DE (1990) Sustained increased cerebral blood flow with prophylactic hypertensive hypervolemic hemodilution ("triple-H-therapy") after subarachnoid hemorrhage. Neurosurgery 27: 729–740

Ostergaard JR, Voldby B (1983) Intracranial arterial aneurysms in children and adolescents. J Neurosurg 58: 832–837

Pakarinen S (1967) Incidence, aetiology and prognosis of primary subarachnoid hemorrhage. Acta Neurol Scand 29: 128

Pandya DN, van Hoesen GW, Mesulam MM (1981) Efferent connections of the cingulate gyrus in the rhesus monkey. Exp Brain Res 42: 319–330

Pardo JV, Pardo PJ, Janer KW, Raichle ME (1990) The anterior cingulate cortex mediates processing selection in the Stroop attentional conflict paradigm. Proc Natl Acad Sci USA 87: 256–259

Parker JW (1957) The validity of some current tests for organicity. J Consult Psychol 21: 425–428

Parkin AJ, Leng NRC, Stanhope N (1988) Memory impairment following ruptured aneurysm of the anterior communicating artery. Brain Cogn 7: 231–243

Parsons OA, Prigatano GP (1978) Methodological considerations in clinical neuropsychological research. J Consult Clin Psychol 46: 608–619

Pendleton M, Heaton R, Lehmann R, Hulihan D (1982) Diagnostic utility of the Thurstone Word Fluency Test in neuropsychological evaluations. J Clin Neuropsychol 4: 307–314

Penrose R, Storey P (1970) Emotional disturbance and subarachnoid haemorrhage. Psychother Psychosom 18: 321–325

Perlmutter D, Rhoton AL (1976) Microsurgical anatomy of the anterior cerebral-anterior communicating-recurrent artery complex. J Neurosurg 45: 259–72

Perneczky A, Koos WT (1982) Special remarks on microsurgical techniques for cerebral aneurysms. Acta Neurochir 63: 101–103

Pfingstmann G, Baumann U (1986) Zur Validierung der FPI-R-Version anhand von Klienten einer Studienberatungsstelle. Z Diff Diagnost Psychol 7: 243–247

Philips LH, Whisnant JP, O'Fallon WM, Sundt TM (1980) The unchanging pattern of subarachnoid hemorrhage in a community. Neurology 30: 1034–1040

Philips S, Sangalang V, Sterns G (1987) Basal forebrain infarction. A clinicopathologic correlation. Arch Neurol 44: 1134–1138

Pool JL (1958) Cerebral vasospasm. N Engl J Med 259: 1259–1264

Porteus SD (1950) The Porteus Maze Test and Intelligence. Palo Alto: Pacific Books

Posner MI, Boies SJ (1972) Components of attention. Psychol Rev 78: 391–408

Posner MI (1982) Cumulative development of attentional theory. Am Psychologist 37: 168–179

Posner MI, Rafal RD (1987) Cognitive theories of attention and the rehabilitation of attentional deficits. In: Meier MJ, Benton AL, Diller L (eds) Neuropsychological rehabilitation. Edinburgh: Churchill Livingstone, pp 86–101

Posner MI, Petersen ST (1990) The attentional system of the human brain. In: Cowan WM, Shooter EM, Stevens CF, Thompson RF (eds) Annual Review of Neuroscience. Vol 13. Palo Alto: Annual Reviews Inc, pp 25–42

Prigatano GP, Wright EL, Levin D (1984) Quality of life and its predictors in patients with mild hypoxemia and chronic obstructive pulmonary disease. Arch Int Med 144: 1613–1619

Prigatano GP (1986) Personality and psychosocial consequences of brain injury. In: Prigatano GP (ed) Neuropsychological rehabilitation after brain injury. Baltimore: Johns Hopkins University Press, pp 29–50

Pritz MB (1991) Evaluation and treatment of aneurysms of the vertebral artery: Different strategies for different lesions. Neurosurgery 29: 247–256

Quincke H (1872) Zur Physiologie der Cerebrospinalflüssigkeit. Arch Anat Physiol: 153–177

Rabinowick AL, Ginsburg DL, DeGiorgio CM, Gott PS, Giannotta SL (1991) Unruptured intracranial aneurysms: seizures and antiepileptic drug treatment following surgery. J Neurosurg 75: 371–373

Rauchfleisch U (1983) Zur Reliabilität und Validität des Aufmerksamkeits-Belastungstests (Test d2) bei Patienten mit hirndiffusem Psychosyndrom und neurotischen Störungen. Diagnostica 24: 247–255

Reulen HJ, Philippon J (1988) Prevention and treatment of delayed ischemic dysfunction in patients with subarachnoid hemorrhage. Acta Neurochir (Suppl) 45

Reul J, Weis J, Spetzger U, Konert T, Fricke C, Thron A (1997) Long-term angiographic and histopathologic findings in experimental aneurysms of the carotid bifurcation embolized with platinum and tungsten coils. Am J Neurol Radiol 18: 35–42

Richardson RT, DeLong MR (1988) A reappraisal of the functions of the nucleus basalis of Meynert. Trends Neurosci 6: 264–267

Richardson JT (1989) Performance in free recall following rupture and repair of intracranial aneurysm. Brain Cogn 9: 210–226

Richardson JT (1991) Cognitive performance following rupture and repair of intracranial aneurysm. Acta Neurol Scand 83: 110–122

Rinkel GJE, van Gijn J, Wijdicks EFM (1993) Subarachnoid hemorrhage without detectable aneurysm. Stroke 24: 1403–1409

Robinson A, Heaton R, Lehman R, Stilson D (1980) The utility of the Wisconsin Card Sorting Test in detecting and localizing frontal lobe lesions. J Consult Clin Psychol 48: 605–614

Robinson RG, Kubos KL, Starr LB, Rao K, Price TR (1984) Mood disorders in stroke patients: Importance of location of lesion. Brain 107: 81–93

Roe H (1852) Aneurism of the anterior cerebral artery. Trans Pathol Soc London 3: 46

Rohde V, Schaller C, Hassler WE (1995) Intraventricular recombinant tissue plasminogen activator for lysis of intraventricular haemorrhage. J Neurol Neurosurg Psychiat 58: 447–451

Rohrmann B (1978) Empirische Studien zur Entwicklung von Antwortskalen für die sozialwissenschaftliche Forschung. Z Sozialpsychol 9: 222–245

Romner B, Sonesson B, Ljunggren B, Brandt L, Säveland H, Holtas S (1989) Late magnetic resonance imaging related to neurobehavioral functioning after aneurysmal subarachnoid hemorrhage. Neurosurgery 25: 390–397

Ropper AH, Zervas NT (1984) Outcome 1 year after SAH from cerebral aneurysm. Management morbidity, mortality and functional status in 112 consecutive good-risk patients. J Neurosurg 60: 909–915

Ruelle A, Lasio G, Boccardo M, Gottlieb A, Severi P (1985) Long-term prognosis of subarachnoid hemorrhage of unknown etiology. J Neurol 232: 277–279

Sahs AL, Perret GE, Locksley HB, Nishioka H (1969) Natural history of subarach noid hemorrhage, intracranial aneurysms and arteriovenous malformations. Based on 6368 cases in the Cooperative Study. In: Locksley HB (ed) Intracranial aneurysms and subarachnoid hemorrhage. A cooperative study. Philadelphia: JB Lippincott, pp 37–108

Samson D, Batjer HH, Bowman G, Mootz L, Krippner WJ, Meyer YJ, Allen BC (1994) A clinical study of the parameters and effects of temporary arterial occlusion in the management of intracranial aneurysm. Neurosurgery 34: 22–29

Sano K, Saito I (1978) Timing and indication of surgery for ruptured intracranial aneurysms with regard to cerebral vasospasm. Acta Neurochir 41: 49–60

Sano H, Kano T, Shinomiya Y (1982) Prospection of chronic vasospasm by CT findings. Acta Neurochir 63: 23–30

Säveland H, Sonesson B, Ljunggren B, Brandt L, Uski T, Zygmont S, Hindfelt B (1986) Outcome evaluation following subarachnoid hemorrhage. J Neurosurg 64: 191–196

Säveland H, Sonesson B, Ljunggren B, Ryman T, Brandt L (1988) Does intravenous nimodipine treatment influence cognition in patients subjected to early aneurysm operation? Acta Neurol Scand 77: 54–59

Säveland H, Hillman J, Brandt L, Edner G, Jakobsson K-E, Algers G (1992) Overall outcome in aneurysmal subarachnoid hemorrhage. J Neurosurg 76: 729–734

Säveland H, Uski T, Sjöholm H, Sonesson B, Brandt L (1996) SPECT with Technetium-99m-HMPAO in relation to late cognitive outcome after surgery for ruptured cerebral aneurysms. Acta Neurochir 138: 301–307

Satzger W, Niedermeier N, Schönberger J, Engel RR, Beck OJ (1995) Timing of operation for ruptured aneurysms and long-term recovery of cognitive functions. Acta Neurochir 136: 168–174

Sbeigh I, Tamas LB, O'Laoire (1986) Epilepsy after operation for aneurysms. Neurosurgery 19: 784–788

Schaller C, Rohde V, Hassler W (1995) Stereotactic puncture and lysis of spontaneous intracerebral hemorrhage using recombinant tissue-plasminogen activator. Neurosurgery 36: 328–333

Scheurer H, Quast A, Richter P, Erbacher H, Kröber HL (1994) Testtheoretische Analyse des Benton Tests aufgrund einer Stichprobe männlicher Gewalttäter. Diagnostica 40: 363–374

Schievink WI, Karemaker JM, Hagemann LM, van der Werf DJM (1989) Circumstances surrounding aneurysmal subarachnoid hemorrhage. Surg Neurol 32: 266–272

Schmidt JU, König F (1986) Untersuchungen zur Validität der revidierten Form des Freiburger Persönlichkeitsinventars FPI-R. Diagnostica 32: 197–208

Schmidt LR, Hacker H, Schwenkmetzger P (1985) Differentialdiagnostische Untersuchungen mit objektiven Persönlichkeitstests und Fragebogen im psychiatrischen Bereich. Diagnostica 31: 22–37

Schorstein J (1944) Carotid ligation in saccular intracranial aneurysms. Br J Surg 28: 50–70

Schramm J, Koht A, Schmidt G, Pechstein U, Taniguchi M, Fahlbusch R (1990) Surgical and electrophysiological observations during clipping of 134 aneurysms with evoked potential monitoring. Neurosurgery 26: 61–70

Schwarz R, Bernhard J, Flechtner H, Küchler T, Hürny C (1990) Lebensqualität in der Onkologie, Vol I. München, Bern, Wien, New York: Zuckschwerdt Verlag

Schwarz R, Bernhard J, Flechtner H, Küchler T, Hürny C (1995) Lebensqualität in der Onkologie, Vol II. München, Bern, Wien, New York: Zuckschwerdt Verlag

Seifert V, Stolke D, Trost HA, Brüning A, Schäffer J (1989a) Incidence, management and outcome of patients with premature rupture of cerebral aneurysms during surgery. In: Frowein RA, Brock M, Klinger M (eds) Advances in neurosurgery, Vol 17. Berlin, Heidelberg, New York: Springer Verlag, pp 203–207

Seifert V, Eisert WG, Stolke D, Goetz C (1989b) Efficacy of single intracisternal bolus injection of recombinant tissue plasminogen activator to prevent delayed cerebral vasospasm after experimental subarachnoid hemorrhage. Neurosurgery 25: 590–598

Seifert V, Trost HA, Stolke D (1990) Management morbidity and mortality in grade IV and V patients with aneurysmal subarachnoid haemorrhage. Acta Neurochir 103: 5–10

Seiler RW, Grolimund P, Aaslid R, Huber P, Nornes H (1986) Cerebral vasospasm evaluated by transcranial ultrasound with clinical grade and CT-visualized subarachnoid hemorrhage. J Neurosurg 64: 594–600

Sengupta RP, Chiu JSP, Brierley H (1975) Quality of survival following direct surgery for anterior communicating artery aneurysms. J Neurosurg 43: 58–64

Shallice T (1982) Specific impairments of planning. In: Broadbent DE, Weiskrantz L (eds) The neuropsychology of cognitive function. London: The Royal Society, pp 199–209

Shapiro AS, Campbell RL, Scully T (1994) Hemorrhagic dilation of the fourth ventricle: an ominous predictor. J Neurosurg 80: 805–809

Shepard RH (1984) Prognosis of spontaneous (nontraumatic) subarachnoid haemorrhage of unknown cause. Lancet 7: 777–778

Shepard RN, Metzler (1971) Mental rotation of three-dimensional objects. Science 171: 701–703

Shoqeirat MA, Mayes A, MacDonald C, Meudell P (1990) Performance on tests sensitive to frontal lobe lesions by patients with organic amnesia: Leng & Parkin revisited. Br J Psychol 29: 401–408

Shoqeirat MA, Mayes AR (1991) Disproportionate incidental spatial-memory and recall deficits in amnesia. Neuropsychologia 8: 749–769

Simonov PV (1986) The emotional brain. New York: Plenum Press

Sinyor D, Jaques P, Kaloupoek DG, Becker R, Goldenberg M, Coopersmith H (1986) Poststroke depression and lesion location: An attempted replication. Brain 109: 537–546

Smith ML, Milner B (1984) Differential effects of frontal lobe lesions on cognitive estimation and spatial memory. Neuropsychologia 22: 697–705

Smith RR, Miller JD (1990) Pathophysiology and clinical evaluation of subarachnoid hemorrhage. In: Youmans JR (ed) Neurological surgery. Philadelphia: Saunders, pp 1644–1660

Sonesson B, Ljunggren B, Säveland H, Brandt L (1987) Cognition and adjustment following late and early surgery for ruptured aneurysms. Neurosurgery 21: 279–287

Sonesson B, Säveland H, Ljunggren B, Brandt L (1989) Cognitive functioning after subarachnoid haemorrhage of unknown origin. Acta Neurol Scand 80: 400–410

Spallone A, Ferrante L, Palatinsky E, Santoro A, Aqui M (1986) Subarachnoid haemorrhage of unknown origin. Acta Neurochir 80: 12–17

Spetzger U, Gilsbach JM (1994) Results of early aneurysm surgery in poor-grade patients. Neurol Res 14: 27–30

Spetzger U, Reul J, Weis J, Bertalanffy H, Thron A, Gilsbach JM (1996) Microsurgically produced bifurcation aneurysms in a rabbit model for endovascular coil embolisation. J Neurosurg 85: 488–495

Spetzger U, Rohde V, Gilsbach JM (1997) Forum: Clips und Coils in der Aneurysmabehandlung. Wien Med Wochenschr 147: 172–177

Spetzger U, Reul J, Thron A, Warnke J, Gilsbach JM (1997) Microsurgical embolectomy and removal of a migrated coil from the middle cerebral artery. Cerebrovasc Dis 7: 226–231

Squire LR (1986) The neuropsychology of memory dysfunction and its assessment. In: Grant I, Adams KM (eds) Neuropsychological assessment of neuropsychiatric disorders. Oxford: Oxford University Press, pp 268–299

Stambrook M, Moore AD, Peters LC, Zubek E, McBeath S, Friesen IC (1991) Head injury and spinal cord injury: differential effects on psychosocial functioning. J Clin Exp Neuropsychol 13: 521–530

Steck P, Beer U, Frey A, Frühschütz HG, Körner A (1990) Testkritische Überprüfung einer 30-Item Version des Visual Retention Tests nach AL Benton. Diagnostica 36: 38–49

Stegen G, Freckmann N (1991) Outcome and rehabilitation after subarachnoid haemorrhage. Zbl Neurochir 52: 37–39

Stehbens WE (1963) Aneurysms and anatomical variations of cerebral arteries. Arch Pathol 75: 45–64

Steiger HJ, Reulen HJ (1986) Low frequency flow fluctuations in saccular aneurysms. Acta Neurochir 83: 131–137

Steiger HJ, Poll A, Liepsch D, Reulen HJ (1987) Haemodynamic stress in lateral saccular aneurysms. Acta Neurochir 86: 86–98

Steiger HJ, Poll A, Liepsch D, Reulen HJ (1988) Haemodynamic stress in terminal aneurysms. Acta Neurochir 93: 18–23

Steinman DR, Bigler ED (1986) Neuropsychological sequelae of ruptured anterior communicating artery aneurysm. Int J Clin Neuropsychol 8: 135–140

Stenhouse LM, Knight RG, Longmore BE, Bishara SN (1991) Long-term cognitive deficits in patients after surgery on aneurysm of the anterior communicating artery. J Neurol Neurosurg Psychiat 54: 909–914

Stolke D, Hoppe B, Seifert V, Rückert N, Dietz H (1987) How good are the results in aneurysm surgery? Psychological aspects of rehabilitation of early and late operated patients with cerebral aneurysm. In: Wüllenweber R, Klinger M, Brock M (eds) Advances in neurosurgery, Vol 15. Berlin, Heidelberg, New York: Springer Verlag, pp 297–301

Stolke D, Seifert V (1992) Single intracisternal bolus of recombinant tissue plasminogen activator in patients with aneurysmal subarachnoid hemorrhage: Preliminary assessment of efficacy and safety in an open clinical study. Neurosurgery 30: 877–881

Storey PB (1967) Psychiatric sequelae of subarachnoid haemorrhage. Br Med J 3: 261–266

Storey PB (1970) Brain damage and personality change after subarachnoid haemorrhage. Br J Psychiat 117: 129–142

Stuss DT, Alexander MP, Liebermann A, Levine H (1978) An extraordinary form of confabulation. Neurology 28: 1166–1172

Stuss DT, Kaplan EF, Benson DF, Weir WS, Chiulli S, Sarazin FF (1982) Evidence for the involvement of orbitofrontal cortex in memory functions: An interference effect. J Comp Physiol Psychol 96: 913–925

Stuss DT, Benson DF (1984) Neuropsychological studies of the frontal lobes. Psychol Bull 95: 3–28

Stuss DT, Ely P, Hugenholz H, Richard T, Larochelle S, Poirier CA, Bell I (1985) Subtle neuropsychological deficits in patients with good recovery after closed head injury. Neurosurgery 17: 41–46

Stuss DT, Benson DF (1986) The frontal lobes. New York: Raven Press

Sundt TM, Whisnant JP (1978) Subarachnoid hemorrhage from intracranial aneurysms. Surgical management and natural history of the disease. N Engl J Med 299: 116–122

Sundt TM, Piepgras DG (1979) Surgical approach to giant intracranial aneurysms. Operative experiences with 80 cases. J Neurosurg 51: 731–742

Sundt TM, Kobayashi S, Fode NC, Whisnant JP (1982) Results and complications of surgical management of 819 intracranial aneurysms in 722 cases. J Neurosurg 56: 753–765

Suzuki J, Yoshimoto T (1973) Early operation for the ruptured intracranial aneurysm. Jpn J Surg 3: 149–156

Suzuki J, Yoshimoto T, Onuma T (1978) Early operation for ruptured intracranial aneurysms – a study of 31 cases operated within the first four days after ruptured aneurysm. Neurol Med Chir 18: 82–89

Suzuki J, Onuma T, Yoshimoto T (1979) Results of early operations on cerebral aneurysms. Surg Neurol 11: 407–412

Sweet WHC (1941) Seeping intracranical aneurysm simulating neoplasm: Syndrome of the corpus callosum. Arch Neurol Psychiatry 45: 86–104

Takaku A, Tanaka S, Mori T, Suzuki J (1979) Postoperative complications in 1.000 cases of intracranial aneurysms. Surg Neurol 12: 137–144

Talland GA (1960) Psychological studies in Korsakoff's psychosis: IV. Memory and learning. J Nerv Ment Dis 130: 366–385

Talland GA (1965) Deranged memory. New York: Academic Press

Talland GA, Sweet WH, Ballantine HT (1967) Amnesic syndrome with anterior communicating artery aneurysm. J Nerv Ment Dis 145: 179–192

Tarachow S (1939) The Korsakoff psychosis in spontaneous subarachnoid hemorrhage. Report on three cases. Am J Psychiat 95: 887–899

Taren JA (1965) Anatomical pathways related to the clinical findings in aneurysms of the anterior communicating artery. J Neurol Neurosurg Psychiat 28: 228–234

Taylor CL, Yuan Z, Selman WR, Ratcheson RA, Rimm AA (1995) Cerebral arterial aneurysm formation and rupture in 20.767 elderly patients: hypertension and other risk factors. J Neurosurg 83: 812–819

Teasdale E (1984) CT scan in severe diffuse head injury: physiological and clinical correlations. J Neurol Neurosurg Psychiat 47: 600–603

Teissier du Cros J, Lhermitte F (1984) Neuropsychological analysis of ruptured saccular aneurysms of the anterior communicating artery after radical therapy. Surg Neurol 22: 353–359

Temkin NR, Dikmen S, Machamer J, McLean A (1989) General versus disease-specific measures: Further work on the Sickness Impact Profile for head injury. Med Care 27: S44–53

Teuber HL (1964) The riddle of frontal lobe function in man. In: Warren JM, Akert JK (eds) The frontal granual cortex and behavior. New York: McGraw-Hill, pp 410–444

Teunissen LL, Rinkel GJE, Algra A, van Gijn J (1996) Risk factors for subarachnoid hemorrhage: A systematic review. Stroke 27: 544–549

Thomas-Anterion C, Duthel R, Dirkx E, Koenig O, Baudoin V, Laurent A, Brunon J (1995) Preservation de la memoire procedurale chez dix-huit patients peres d'un aneurisme de l'artere communicante anterieure. Neurochirurgie 42: 54–60

Thompson JG (1988) The psychobiology of emotions. New York: Plenum Press

Thorbecke R (1994) Lebensqualität bei Menschen mit schwerer Epilepsie. Epilepsie-Blätter 7: 3–12

Tidswell P, Dias PS, Sagar HJ, Mayes AR, Battersby RDE (1995) Cognitive outcome after aneurysm rupture: relationship to aneurysm site and perioperative complications. Neurology 45: 875–882

Tokuda Y, Inagawa T, Katho Y, Kumano K, Ohbayashi N, Yoshioka H (1995) Intracerebral hematoma in patients with ruptured cerebral aneurysms. Surg Neurol 43: 272–277

Tooth CL, Hadjiivassiliou M, Romanowski C, Byrne J, Oxbury S, Battersby RD, Mayes AR, Sagar HJ (1997) A comparison of cognitive outcome and structural damage following neurosurgical or endovascular treatment of aneurysmal subarachnoid haemorrhage. In: Hütter BO, Gilsbach JM (eds) Neuropsychology in neurosurgery, psychiatry and neurology. Aachen: Augustinus Verlag, pp 85–86

Troupp H, Björksten G (1981) Results of a controlled trial of late surgical versus conservative treatment of intracranial arterial aneurysms. J Neurosurg 35: 20–24

Tsementzis SA, Kennet RP, Hitchcock ER, Gill JS, Beevers DG (1991) Seasonal variation of cerebrovascular disease. Acta Neurochir 111: 80–83

TÜV-Baden MPI (1976) Testnormen für das Wiener Determinationsgerät. Freiburg: TÜV Baden

Uzell BP, Langfitt TW, Dolinskas CA (1987) Influence of injury severity on quality of survival after head injury. Surg Neurol 27: 419–429

Uzell BP (1988) Quality of survival after head injury. Surg Neurol 29: 246–247

Van Dam FSA, Aaronson AK (1988) Quality of life and treatment for Cancer. J Drug Ther Res 13: 173–175

Van der Linden M, Bruyer R, Roland J, Schils JP (1993) Proactive interference in patients with amnesia resulting from anterior communicating artery aneurysm. J Clin Exp Neuropsychol 15: 525–536

Van Gijn J, Hijdra A, Wijdicks EFM, Vermeulen M, van Crevel H (1985a) Acute hydrocephalus after subarachnoid hemorrhage. J Neurosurg 63: 355–362

Van Gijn J, Van Dongen KJ, Vermeulen M, Hijdra A (1985b) Perimesencephalic hemor rhage: a nonaneurysmal and benign form of subarachnoid hemorrhage. Neurology 35: 493–497

Van Zomeren AH, Brower WH, Deelman BG (1984) Attentional deficits: The riddles of selectivity, speed and alertness. In: Brooks DH (ed) Psychological deficits after head injury. New York, Oxford: Oxford University Press, pp 132–149

Van Zomeren AH, Brouwer WH (1987) Head injury and concepts of attention. In: Levin HS, Grafman J, Eisenberg HM (eds) Neurobehavioral recovery from head injury. New York, Oxford: Oxford University Press, pp 398–415

Vassilouthis J, Richardson AE (1979) Ventricular dilatation and communicating hydrocephalus following spontaneous subarachnoid hemorrhage. J Neurosurg 51: 341–351

Vickrey BG, Hays RD, Herman BP, Bladin PF, Batzel LW (1993) Outcomes with respect to quality of life. In: Engel J (ed) Surgical treatment of epilepsies, 2nd ed. New York: Raven Press, pp 623–635

Viefhues H (1991) Quality of life: Semantic history, political and scientific terminology, measurement and methodology, medical research. In: Viefhues H, Schoene W, Rychlik R (eds) Chronic heart failure. Berlin, Heidelberg, New York: Springer, pp 66–91

Vilkki J (1985) Amnesic syndromes after surgery of anterior communicating artery aneurysms. Cortex 21: 431–444

Vilkki J, Holst P, Öhman J, Servo A, Heiskanen O (1989) Cognitive deficits related to computed tomographic findings after surgery for a ruptured intracranial aneurysm. Neurosurgery 26: 579–585

Vilkki J, Holst P, Öhman J, Servo A, Heiskanen O (1990) Social outcome related to cognitive performance and computed tomographic findings after surgery for a ruptured intracranial aneurysm. Neurosurgery 26: 579–585

Vincentelli F, Lehman G, Caruso G, Grisoli F, Rabehanta P, Gouaze A (1991) Extracerebral course of the perforating branches of the anterior communicating artery: Microsurgical anatomy study. Surg Neurol 35: 98–104

Visser MC, van Kooten F, Koudstaal PJ, Passchier J, Grobbee DE, van Gijn J (1996) Quality of life after an ischemic stroke. Cerebrovasc Dis 6: S30

Volpe BT, Hirst (1983) Amnesia following the rupture and repair of an anterior communicating artery aneurysm. J Neurol Neurosurg Psychiat 46: 704–709

Volpe BT, Herscovitch P, Raichle ME (1984) Positron emission tomography defines metabolic abnormity in mesial temporal lobes of two patients with amnesia after rupture and repair of anterior communicating artery aneurysm. Neurology 34: S188

Von Cramon D, Ziehl J (1989) Neuropsychologische Rehabilitation. Grundlagen-Diagnostik-Behandlungsverfahren. Berlin, Heidelberg, New York, Wien: Springer

Von Cramon DY, Mai N, Ziegler W (1995) Neuropsychologische Diagnostik. London, Weinheim: Chapman & Hall

Wallesch CW, Kornhuber, HH, Köllner C, Lücking C (1983) Language and cognitive deficits resulting from medial and dorsolateral frontal lobe lesions. Arch Psychiat 233: 279–296

Walsh KW (1987) Neuropsychology: A clinical approach, 2nd ed. New York: Churchill Livingstone

Walton JN (1953) The Korsakow syndrome in spontaneous subarachnoid hemorrhage. J Ment Sci 99: 521–530

Walton D (1958) The diagnostic and predictive accuracy of the Wechsler Memory Scale in psychiatric patients over 65. J Ment Sci 104: 1111–1118

Wang P, Kaplan J, Rogers E (1975) Memory functioning in hemiplegics: a neuropsychological analysis of the Wechsler Memory Scale. Arch Phys Med Rehabil 56: 517–521

Ware JE (1984) Conceptualizing disease impact and treatment outcome. Cancer 153: 2316–2323

Wassmann H, Werner C, Stockert A (1989) Temporary vessel occlusion by microvascular clips. In: Frowein RA, Brock M, Klinger M (eds) Advances in neurosurgery. Vol 17. Berlin, Heidelberg, New York: Springer Verlag, pp 208–213

Webster JE, Gurdijan ES, Lindner DW, Hardy WG (1960) Proximal occlusion of the anterior cerebral artery. Arch Neurol 2: 19–26

Weir B (1993) The surgical management of anterior circulation aneurysms. Neurosurg Q 1: 19–28

Weisberg LA (1985) Ruptured aneurysm of anterior cerebral or anterior communicating arteries: CT patterns. Neurology 35: 1562–1566

WFNS (1988) WFNS scale of SAH classification. J Neurosurg 68: 985–986

WHO (1980) International classification of impairments, disabilities, and handicaps. Genf: World Health Organisation

Wichern H (1911) Zur Diagnose perforierender Aneurysmen der Hirnarterien. Münch Med Wochenschr 58: 2724–2729

Winn HR, Almaani WS, Berga SL, Jane JA, Richardson AE (1983) The long term outcome in patients with multiple aneurysms – incidence of late hemorrhage and implications of incidental aneurysms. J Neurosurg 59: 642–651

Wiseman R (1676) Several chirurgicall treatises. London: R Royston & B Took

Yasargil MG, Fox JL, Ray MW (1975) The operative approach to aneurysm of the anterior communicating artery. In: Krayenbühl H (ed) Advances and technical standards in neurosurgery. Vol II. Wien, New York: Springer Verlag, pp 115–128

Yasargil MG (1984) Microneurosurgery. Vol II. Stuttgart, New York: Thieme Verlag

Yates JW, Chalmer B, McKegney P (1980) Evaluation of patients with advanced cancer using the Karnofsky Performance scale. Cancer 145: 2220–2224

Zimmermann P, Fimm B (1992) Testbatterie zur Aufmerksamkeitsprüfung (TAP) Version 1.02. Würselen: Psytest Verlag

Zubrick S, Smith A (1978) Factors affecting BVRT performance in adults with acute focal cerebral lesions. Paper presented at the sixth International Neuropsychological Society meeting in Minneapolis